'It is always refreshing to deal with a differer
hygienic exercise. Michael's knowledge of an
Health Wand make him unique in the Tai Chi
congratulated in making this rare material avail
every success.'

— *Dan Docherty, Chairman of the Tai Chi Union for Great Britain, UK*

'We have more and more need in these frenetic times for the wisdom of Chinese medicine. Michael shows very clearly how Jiangan exercises can be used to benefit ourselves. I regularly see, in my own practice, how people's health and vitality can be transformed by following such exercise regimes. I can wholeheartedly recommend this book for those who want to become more healthy and for those who want to maintain their health.'

— *Dr Stephen Gascoigne, medical doctor, acupuncturist and herbalist, UK and Ireland*

JIANGAN
THE CHINESE
HEALTH
WAND

of related interest

Eternal Spring
Taijiquan, Qi Gong, and the Cultivation of Health, Happiness and Longevity
Michael W. Acton
ISBN 978 1 84819 003 0

Managing Stress with Qigong
Gordon Faulkner
Foreword by Carole Bridge
ISBN 978 1 84819 035 1

The Yang Tàijí 24-Step Short Form
A Step-by-Step Guide for all Levels
James Drewe
ISBN 978 1 84819 041 2

You Are How You Move
Experiential Chi Kung
Ged Sumner
ISBN 978 1 84819 014 6

JIANGAN
THE CHINESE
HEALTH
WAND

Michael Davies

SINGING
DRAGON

LONDON AND PHILADELPHIA

The photographs in the book have been kindly provided by Rob Purbrick of Purpix Media and Photography (www.purpix.co.uk)

First published in 2011
by Singing Dragon
an imprint of Jessica Kingsley Publishers
116 Pentonville Road
London N1 9JB, UK
and
400 Market Street, Suite 400
Philadelphia, PA 19106, USA

www.singingdragon.com

Library of Congress Cataloging in Publication Data
Davies, Michael.
  Jiangan-- the Chinese health wand / Michael Davies.
    p. cm.
  ISBN 978-1-84819-077-1 (alk. paper)
  1. Wand exercises. 2. Exercise therapy. 3. Health. 4. Medicine, Chinese.
  I. Title.
  GV503.D38 2011
  613.7'1--dc22
                          2011012108

British Library Cataloguing in Publication Data
A CIP catalogue record for this book is available from the British Library

ISBN 978 1 84819 077 1

Printed and bound in Great Britain

Contents

1

Discovering the 'Chinese Wand Exercise' (Jiangan)

While visiting Malaysia in 1981 I stayed at a cut-price 'chalet' on the East Coast, a ramshackle building I shared with backpackers. My surroundings were certainly austere but had I the financial resources to stay in the nearby luxury hotel, I would have missed the opportunity to witness a nightly demonstration of a rare art. Each evening before the elderly Chinese caretaker brought out his camp bed to sleep in the little foyer of our building, I watched him perform a series of exercises with a bamboo pole about the length of a broom handle. He moved slowly and gracefully, bending, twisting, keeping the pole close to his body but sometimes circling and spiralling it around his head. At the time I had just begun learning Taiji (which is another word for Tai Chi) and so guessed that I was witnessing some form of internal Chinese exercise. I scribbled some hasty functional drawings of the old man's movements and showed my Taiji teacher on my return to London, who solved the mystery by producing a book titled *Chinese Wand Exercise* by Bruce L. Johnson,[1] the American who discovered the obscure set of exercises in Shanghai in 1945.

In the summer of 2009 while attending several Taiji and Qigong seminars, it struck me that most of these events – and indeed most martial

---

1   Johnson, B.L. (1977) *Chinese Wand Exercise.* New York: Morrow.

arts classes – begin with general warm-ups, stretching and breathing exercises that seem numerous but rather random. I wondered, half-seriously, whether a combined warm-up, stretching and breathing routine could be devised that was not only safe for beginners and advanced practitioners alike but also comprehensive in range and effect, consistent and based on scientific and logical sequence. This would certainly be a tall order. Yet according to a book gathering dust on my bookshelf for years, such a system has existed as long as Chinese civilisation itself. The book, one of many obscure titles on Chinese martial arts and philosophy I inherited from my teacher, was, of course, the *Chinese Wand Exercise*. Over the years I had only occasionally taken it from the bookshelf and flicked through the pages with mild interest. To be honest, the photos of exercises performed with a bamboo pole looked so formidable and challenging that I was hesitant to try them. But finally reading the book from cover to cover, it became clear that I had found the perfect warm-up and stretching routine for my own Taiji class. I was particularly intrigued by Johnson's claim that the system was the best exercise ever devised. Like many Taiji practitioners, I had always regarded Taiji as filling that role, but sometimes we need to re-evaluate long-held practices and beliefs, so I became a 'student of the Wand' to test Johnson's claim. Over the following months I practised the Wand exercises diligently each day, using a wooden staff of the dimensions directed by Johnson and following his instructions to the letter. My research convinced me that regular practice of this art can produce the wonderful health benefits associated with internal health systems such as Yoga, Qigong and Taiji. I also realised that the Chinese Wand Exercise can be practised as a health system in its own right and has a unique methodology and philosophy. In fact, it has the potential to be more effective than any other type of daily exercise. Support for this extraordinary claim not only comes from the decades of anecdotal evidence from Johnson's students and my own experience but also can be logically deduced from the practices and methodology of the system.

Although these ancient exercises have much in common with Yoga, Qigong and Taiji, the main difference is that the complexity and depth of these other Eastern arts reflect their multifaceted aims, whether it be spiritual development, martial skill or healing specific internal organs. The Chinese Wand Exercise, which dates back many centuries – perhaps thousands of years – was created to be a simple but effective daily exercise regime that anyone can perform, a sort of 'Royal Canadian Air Force System' of the ancient world,[2] and has been subjected to centuries of development, trial and error and adaptation to reach a state of near perfection. It is true to say that other ancient Eastern systems have developed simplified exercise routines for everyday practice but only comparatively recently, so in the context of a *daily regime* they are not as 'tried and tested' as the Chinese Wand Exercise. So what precisely are these exercises? Exercises can be split into two types: 'external' and vigorous programmes that cannot be practised every day due to the danger of muscle fatigue and strain, and 'internal' or therapeutic (sometimes called 'mind-body') exercises like Yoga, Taiji and Qigong which develop the inner self and can be practised every day of one's life without any ill effects. These internal or mind-body systems are part of our healthy daily regime, along with bathing and eating nutritious food, and can be considered 'nutrition' for the body. The Chinese Wand Exercise certainly falls into this category. However, the system is also capable of delivering the body-shaping and conditioning effects associated with more physically robust exercises such as gym work. The ability to perform body-changing exercises every day without sore muscles or strain is a great advantage for those looking to lose weight or tone muscles. This remarkable feat is largely achieved by using the unique methodology of splitting each posture into graduated stages, each with its own breathing cycle, which prepares the muscles by gradually stretching them to minimise stress and strain. This makes the system probably the safest in existence. After we finish a session we do not feel tired or exhausted but energised, fresh and alert. The art's deep diaphragmatic breathing and easy-to-learn simple-to-practise movements form an integrated and complete daily maintenance regime. Muscles are strengthened and stretched gently, joints are opened and kept supple, the cardiovascular system is stimulated, blood circulation is improved and meditative focus relieves tension and activates the body's healing energies. The exercises emphasise control, precision, centring the body, deep breathing and focus in mind and body. Movements are never performed rapidly or repeated excessively; instead, the focus is

---

2   A system of exercise created in the late 1950s for the purpose of keeping the average person, including sedentary workers, fit and healthy.

on gradual advancement and quality of movement, not quantity. The low impact nature makes it ideal for injury prevention and rehabilitation. The movements also precision-train the body to move efficiently with minimal impact on the body, which helps us relax even in the midst of a stressed environment. People take up internal mind-body exercises to feel more energetic, happier and more peaceful. But in the case of the Chinese Wand Exercise, 'fitter' and 'slimmer' can be added to the list.

When I researched the history of the Chinese Wand Exercise, I found almost nothing that was not mentioned in Johnston's book. The system, it seems, is forgotten in China, though I have often wondered if there are any masters still practising the art in a remote region. Even the phrase 'Chinese Wand Exercise' reminds us of an orphan hastily renamed after arriving in the West; so for serious study I thought that a Chinese name was desirable, if only out of respect for the culture from which it came. With the help of some Chinese friends, I found a term used for a collection of obscure games of strength with a pole.[3] Although there is no apparent link with these games, the name 'Jiangan' (健杆) is accurately descriptive for the Chinese Wand Exercise. It is pronounced *Jee-en Gan* and means 'health stick' or 'health pole'. In this book the term 'Gan' will be used for 'Wand' and 'Jiangan' will replace 'Chinese Wand Exercise'.

Soon after I began using Jiangan for warm-ups in my own Taiji classes, it became obvious that it had more to offer, so I now also promote it as a complete daily exercise as it was originally intended. In particular, it is invaluable for those who want to learn a mind-body health system but who find the many types on offer difficult to master. Jiangan's greatest advantage is that it is quite easy to learn.

I was urged by friends to write a small book with instructions on how to perform the exercises, but from this initial objective the project has expanded to encompass the philosophy and methodology behind the art. In particular I found significant parallels between Jiangan and Chinese philosophy and even discovered esoteric and philosophical perspectives from ancient Egypt. Therefore not only is Jiangan a fascinating addition to Chinese internal

---

3 Described as a 'health bar' (健杆) and devised by people in Jing Ning She Autonomous County in ZheJiang Province, East China.

health arts but also it could be a key to understanding ancient mind-body philosophy from the dawn of humankind.

The primary objective of this book is to introduce Jiangan to practitioners of the internal arts and encourage them to use it as an all-round conditioner and warm-up for class. But it is hoped that many will also take it up as a stand-alone health system.

2

History

The 'history' of Jiangan is essentially the remarkable story of one American's discovery of a Chinese treasure. In 1945, a group of young US sailors disembarked from their ship anchored in Shanghai harbour to take in the sights of the famous city. They hired a large rickshaw then sat back in amazement as the thin elderly driver sped away carrying five burly sailors – amounting to over a thousand pounds in weight. Noticing that the driver's pace did not let up even on sharp inclines and that he did not seem to get breathless, the strongest sailor, navy wrestling champion Bruce L. Johnson, was so intrigued that he changed places with the driver to see how he would fare pulling the full rickshaw. He was unable to negotiate inclines and quickly became breathless. Each sailor tried but failed to match the feat of the elderly driver. Johnson, who at that young age was something of a fitness fanatic and 'strongman' who used to entertain the ship's company with gymnastic feats, was determined to discover the source of the driver's strength. After making enquiries he was soon introduced to Dr Cheng, Jiangan master.

Dr Cheng claimed to be 93 years old, but Johnson observed that he resembled a man in his fifties. After a humbling demonstration of the elderly man's superior strength by way of a friendly bout of sparring, Johnson was left in no doubt that what he had always regarded as 'strength' and 'fitness' were inferior to the source of Dr Cheng's vitality. When Dr Cheng realised that the young American was serious about health and fitness, he showed him the many bamboo poles placed all around his house like revered instruments. These 'Gan', or 'Wands' as Johnson called them, were very impressive, with carvings and inscriptions in Chinese characters. Many were additionally ingrained with pieces of copper (which Dr Cheng explained was a natural conductor of 'life force'). Some bamboo Gan looked exceptionally old and had, Dr Cheng claimed, belonged to practitioners who had died many years earlier. So logically, if Dr Cheng was 93 at the time, we can say with a degree of confidence that Jiangan must have been in existence at least in the early 1800s. However, Dr Cheng maintained that the art was thousands of years old.

This is a short synopsis of the history. Jiangan had its origins in a type of weight training involving primitive barbells made from bamboo poles with stones attached. Eventually the weights were discarded and the pole used to align and guide the body in a series of more subtle movements combined with breathing. By the time of the early emperors, there had been many centuries of observation, trial, error and experimentation, and these exercises were deemed suitable for court physicians to teach the Imperial family. But can we take this history at face value? After all, many Chinese martial arts and esoteric systems claim Imperial patronage that adds a 'cultural kudos' to the lineage. Common legends involve sages in possession of miraculous health systems that so impress an emperor that he adopts them and keeps them as a secret to be passed down within the Imperial family. Of course, these stories cannot all be true. Even if a particular emperor was so enamoured with an esoteric practice or a martial art and studied it diligently for hours each day, it is unlikely that members of his family and future generations would be equally enthusiastic to devote hours a day to its study. Therefore, Jiangan, being comparatively simple to practise, offers a more plausible scenario of Imperial exercise regimes. It is easy to imagine a daily exercise programme administered by royal physicians in a similar way that famous people today have their personal trainers and nutritionists. The scene is set in a courtyard in the palace where the Imperial family are taken through a daily routine of Jiangan, the art that is simple, easy to learn and requires little enthusiasm for esoteric concepts.

At some stage Imperial patronage ended and Jiangan experts were scattered across China, keeping the perfected art as family secrets. So we arrive in 1945 and Dr Cheng, having lost both his sons in the Sino-Japanese war and with no one to carry on the art, entrusted a young American to take the secrets of Jiangan overseas. If Dr Cheng had not done so and Johnson had not written his book, the art would undoubtedly have been lost forever. It is staggering how many internal cultivation exercises exist in China. Even today, it is not too rare an occurrence for Chinese academics to discover scrolls or ancient documents revealing a hitherto unknown style of Qigong or martial art. This raises the question: how many ingenious mind-body systems have been lost in China? Passing down knowledge to future generations is a perilous process, especially if it also has to be kept a secret, as so many Chinese systems invariably were. It is not known whether the instructions for Jiangan were ever written down at any point in Chinese history, and perhaps one day an old document will be discovered complete with drawings. It is more likely that the system was passed on by word of mouth, which makes it all the more remarkable that it survived at all.

In the mid-1970s the 'Chinese Wand Exercise' was poised to sweep the USA as Bruce Johnson, the young sailor who had diligently mastered the system, promoted the art in a manner that Dr Cheng would approve of. Johnson stressed its unique qualities and superiority over the exercises practised in the West, such as aerobics and isometrics, and also warned – decades before sports trainers came to the same conclusion – that the exercises taught in schools and colleges were potentially harmful. He also wanted the exercises to be promoted by doctors, hospitals, nursing homes and educational establishments. He was also astute enough to realise the parallel between modern Western lifestyle and Chinese Imperial families: the consumption of rich food, excessive alcohol, lethargy, obesity, overeating, inaction, all were factors which the exercise system had been designed to combat centuries earlier in an efficient yet accessible way. In particular he stressed Jiangan's astounding weight-reducing capabilities, which hit a chord in US consumer society. Various newspaper articles reported how quickly some people dropped their clothes size after just a few sessions with the 'Wand' and it was undoubtedly the 'shed inches and pounds with the Chinese Wand' catchphrase that propelled Johnson onto the famous Dinah Shore TV talk show. As an instructor and fitness consultant at Paramount Studios, he attracted celebrity students such as Clint Walker and James Coburn, then he served as adviser and critic for the US Government body the President's Council on Physical Fitness, where he continued promoting the art as 'the most superior exercise system ever devised'. When he published his book in 1977, it became a great success and sold throughout the world; and so the wishes of Dr Cheng to make Jiangan known to the wider population came to fruition.

Yet even though the art arrived in the West many decades before Taiji and Qigong, it ultimately failed to make the breakthrough into the mainstream. For all the media hype on weight loss, Johnson did not market it on a large scale, preferring to teach in small numbers at his home. This could be the reason why Jiangan has been confined to semi-obscurity for decades. Although there are still many classes throughout the USA that approach it the way Johnson taught, it is often presented as a sort of 'quirky physical exercise to improve posture or balance' or even combined with aerobics or some other hybrid fitness class. Yet it is clear from Johnson's book that Dr Cheng taught the art as a branch of internal Chinese health, and this approach is essential to obtain all the potent health benefits that remain hidden in the system like gems. Treating Jiangan as an internal Chinese art will also allow us to understand its unique philosophical and metaphysical qualities.

3

The Gan Itself

Trial and error over the ages has produced the perfect Gan – between 1.22m and 1.27m (48" to 50") in length and between 2.5cm and 2.8cm (1" to 1⅛") in diameter. The Gan should be as light as possible to avoid putting undue strain on the body. This is because Jiangan is not a type of weight lifting and should not be confused with exercises using weighted bars. Weight training was abandoned very early on by the masters because it tires the body instead of rejuvenating it. A heavy Gan also makes the movements more difficult to perform and can result in fatigue and strains, which are the very things we seek to avoid. Bamboo is the perfect material to use because it is both light and strong and produces just the right amount of resistance. Because of its ready availability in China and its association with Chinese internal arts, it is the perfect material for a Gan. Many people say that bamboo has a special quality and they feel in touch with nature itself when they hold an object made of bamboo, experiencing a fascinating almost 'magical' aspect, as if it has an individual personality. No matter how identically measured and cut, no two bamboo Gans are alike either in look, feel or weight. When I received my first batch of bamboo poles from China, I was amazed how each of them, despite being within the required dimensions, felt quite different.

You can use wooden dowels but they are heavier than bamboo and as you go through the exercises, those extra grams make all the difference. Ideally,

Gan should be under 300 grams, though many bamboo Gan I have used have been considerably lighter.

It is very much a matter of personal taste which Gan we choose to be our own. Traditionally in China the process of choosing a Gan is thought to have been one of great importance and we can ascertain from the careful practice of choosing bamboo flutes that a similar process took place with Jiangan masters. A person would handle many 'raw' bamboo poles until one was found that has the right 'feel' or 'energy' for that individual. It is said that a Gan eventually reflects the energy of its owner and when such a bond has been developed over many years, another person even touching the object destroys the 'power of accumulated energy'.

If you decide to begin with a wooden dowel, I would not suggest using a conventional broom handle as the dimensions are not likely to be correct for the average person. Most are much too short and many are much too thick. In particular there must be *no* compromise in the length, since it is this that gives Jiangan its special qualities. Just why this particular length is so important has been a mystery for many years but I believe the secret is in the ratio of the Gan length to the height of the human body.

THE GOLDEN SECTION

Leonardo Fibonacci, the man who introduced Arabic numerals to the West in the twelfth century, discovered a series of numbers that are created by adding the sum of the preceding two numbers:

1	1	2	3	5	8	13	21	34
		1+1=2	1+2=3	2+3=5	3+5=8	5+8=13	8+13=21	13+21=34

When we divide one number in the series with the number before it, we obtain numbers very close to one another:

$13 \div 8 = 1.625$

$34 \div 21 = 1.619$

After the thirteenth in the series the number tends to round to 1.618 – the Golden Ratio.

In fact, the Golden Ratio was known in ancient times and Pythagoras (c.560–c.480 BC), the Greek mathematician and philosopher, proved that it was the basis for the proportions of the human figure. He showed that the human body is built with each part in a definite *Golden Proportion* to all the other parts. His discoveries had a tremendous influence on Greek art. Every part of their major buildings, down to the smallest detail of decoration, was constructed upon this proportion. The proportions of the human body are also set out according to the Golden Ratio. When the distance between the foot and navel is regarded as a unit, then the height of a human equals 1.618 of this unit. This is 'φ' (phi), or 1.618, the Golden Ratio. It can be found not only in all external aspects of the human body but also in internal organs. It has been positively identified in lung structure and the inner ear, but most significantly in the structure of DNA itself. The length of the curve in each helix of a DNA molecule is 34 angstroms and the width is 21 angstroms.[1] In the Fibonacci series 21 and 34 are consecutive numbers: $34 \div 21 = 1.619$. The Golden Ratio is well represented in biology. Once an egg is fertilised it divides and multiplies in number until it reaches a point at which the ratio of the succeeding number of cells to the previous number of cells is phi, 1.618. There is no reason to believe that the Golden Ratio does not go further and it seems as if we are programmed with it in every part of our being.

What has all this to do with the length of the Gan? Since the old masters were so adamant about its length, I wondered whether this had something to do with its ratio to the human body. First, I took the height of the Gan and my own height and noted the position of the Gan against my body. For simplicity I defined my body's height as '13' to show the ratio more easily within the Fibonacci series (Figure I). The tip of the Gan came up to one of the Golden Ratio points that the body can be split into if measured from the top of the head (line '3' in Figure II). This should be the case with everybody. If you hold the Gan vertically next to your body, the end should come up to your upper chest around the height of your armpit. I then measured my arms; they are 30 inches long. My Gan is 50 inches long: $50 \div 30 = 1.666$, which means that the Gan is roughly the Golden Ratio of the length of my arms, and this seems to be the secret behind the Gan's length (Figure III). Although no two people's arms are the same length, the general ratio of the Gan to

---

1   An angstrom is a unit of measurement: one ten-millionth of a millimetre, or 1×10^{-10} metres.

the arms will be around 1.618. What this discovery gives us is a measure for the length of Gan suitable for people of different heights, including children. There is no need to be too precise, but the figure we should be aiming for when calculating the ratio of arm length to Gan is around 1.6.

Was the length of the Gan chosen deliberately after consideration of the Golden Ratio or did the masters feel naturally in tune with the Golden Ratio? Whichever it is, practitioners of the art soon discover that the particular length of the Gan provides an energised effect whereas other lengths do not.

To find the correct length Gan for short people and children, there is a simple test. Place the Gan with one end on the floor next to the person; it should come up to about the top of the person's armpit (or comfortably fit inside the armpit); see Figures II and III for the general range. There is some degree of leeway of course, and an inch or two either way is not of great importance. But if the Gan comes up above the shoulder it is definitely too long and a shorter Gan will be needed. If you are sure that this is the case, you can cut a Gan to size. In my experience a 50 inch Gan should be adequate for the tallest long-armed person, but there will be exceptions – very tall people will require Gan a few inches longer than the norm.

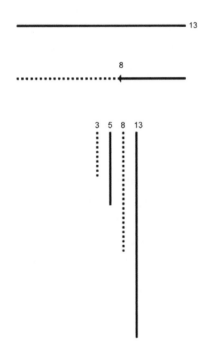

Figure I

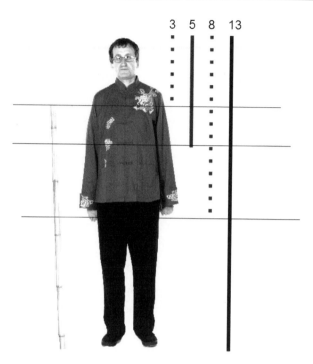

Figure II

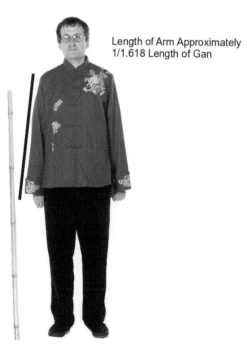

Length of Arm Approximately
1/1.618 Length of Gan

Figure III

OBTAINING GAN

It will probably be easier to find a wooden Gan to begin with. Local hardware shops, DIY stores and lumber yards sell wooden poles of various lengths and correct thickness which can be cut to size. In particular, you can obtain longer handles for brooms and mops from these outlets, as ordinary broom and mop handles will probably be too short.

Why not make your own Gan? You could follow the lead of people who make hiking staves or walking staffs from suitable straight tree branches. To get the 'feel' of the exercises you can even improvise a Gan out of various everyday objects. Curtain or shower rails or strong cardboard tubes of the correct thickness may be suitable in the short term, but make sure that they are not flexible or too heavy – and, of course, that they can be cut to the correct length. If you want a bamboo Gan, garden centres sell a range of bamboo poles but it may be difficult to find the exact size. Again, you could cut longer bamboo to the correct length and start with a slightly thinner pole, as these are more abundant. If you wish to practise with a bamboo Gan of the correct dimensions you will probably have to obtain bamboo poles that are specially cut and imported.

There are many companies importing bamboo poles from their natural habitat overseas, especially from East Asia, but I have found that it is difficult to obtain the exact dimensions needed. The UK Wand Initiative (www.jiangan.org), an organisation set up to promote Jiangan, imports good quality bamboo Gan of the correct dimensions from reliable suppliers in China and keeps a supply in stock. These bamboo poles are lacquered with a light varnish to preserve them, and will last a lifetime.

4

Philosophy

ANIMAL OBSERVATION

Like all Chinese internal arts, Jiangan is influenced by ancient Chinese philosophy and one of the unique long-standing themes is taking a lead from the animal kingdom in the way of behaviour and living. In Yang style Taiji, there are postures named after animals moving in a particular way, such as 'Snake Creeps Down' and 'White Crane Spreads its Wings'. In Qigong there is a famous routine called 'Five Animal Frolics', which follows the distinctive movements of certain animals. More ancient Qigong has stances named after the bear, eagle, turtle, monkey, leopard, chicken, horse, cobra and praying mantis. Whether it is the superficial look of a posture or the quality of movement that is stressed, animals are of great importance in Chinese internal health systems. In Jiangan there are also postures named after animals, including 'Stretching the Crane', 'Twisting the Snake' and 'The Rocking Bear', but the animal influence is also more philosophical. The old masters took the principles of natural living of the animal kingdom and observed that the daily lives of animals can be split into three parts:

- Hunting-gathering (survival activities).

- Eating, drinking, sleeping, toilet, etc. (body function activities).

- Playing-exercising (development and maintenance activities).

When one of these areas is disrupted, the other areas tend to be affected. For example, domesticated animals who do not hunt or gather tend to overeat, become lazy, fail to exercise and develop illnesses they would not have in the wild. Humans also follow this threefold pattern of life and when one important area is removed from the cycle the whole system can collapse. The Chinese Imperial family were, in effect, domesticated animals who did not work or exercise and therefore lived unbalanced lives. Jiangan brought back their life balance by daily exercise focused on countering their sedentary state.

DAOISM

In his instructions to Bruce Johnson, Dr Cheng talked of energy stored at the base of the spine rising to the top of the head and referred to the Gan 'recirculating Qi around the body to prevent it dissipating'. This is the language of Daoist philosophy and affirms that Jiangan belongs to Chinese internal medicine. The concept of Qi '气' is one of the most profound and difficult aspects of Chinese philosophy to explain. It has came to mean 'energy', 'breath' or 'vapour', and as far as Jiangan is concerned Qi has two qualities – 'Heavenly Qi', which manifests in nature and 'Human Qi', which exists within the human body. Human Qi fluctuates because of worldly endeavours, illness and other factors and the body becomes deficient in Qi or its 'flow' is blocked. So humans are dependent on Heavenly Qi, which does not need to be replenished. Chinese internal medicine seeks to replenish Qi and stimulate its flow in the body through pathways called meridians via exercises or acupuncture. Qigong is the best known method of exercise; Taiji is another way – and so is Jiangan.

Yin and Yang

The concept of 'Yin' and 'Yang' is arguably the most important in Chinese internal arts and is one of the fundamental principles in Jiangan. The original state before the universe was known as 'Wuji' (無極) meaning 'without ridge-pole', which was interpreted as 'limitless void' and often represented by an empty circle. From Wuji comes Taiji (太極) meaning 'great extremes or polarities', which consists of two opposing forces, Yin (阴) and

Yang (阳), each becoming their opposite when they reach the extreme point. As well as being represented by the famous Yin-Yang symbol (a circle with two 'embryos'), the Yin and Yang concept can also be depicted with broken and unbroken lines (see Figure IV). Not only does the slow regular breathing employed in Jiangan emphasise the alternation from Yin to Yang, but also each exercise is built upon the Yin-Yang principle.

The Five Elements

The alternation of Yin and Yang generates the 'Five Phases of Qi', more popularly known as the Five Elements – earth, metal, water, wood and fire (also in Figure IV). These Five Elements are also important in Jiangan because each exercise is split into several parts, each corresponding to an element.

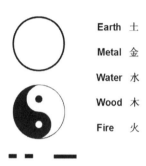

Earth　土

Metal　金

Water　水

Wood　木

Fire　　火

Figure IV

Qi Balance in the Body

Jiangan stresses the concept that everyone is made up of 'Yin Qi' and 'Yang Qi' and an imbalance of either causes illness, and so like all branches of traditional Chinese medicine, Jiangan aims to keep a balance of Yin and Yang in the body. Yang Qi is like fire. It heats you up. An excess and you are prone to temper and tension. It also gears you up for dangerous situations and the stresses of the world – rather like adrenalin. Deficiency in Yang Qi means that you feel 'run down', sluggish, with a general lack of energy. An excess of Yang Qi 'burns up' Yin Qi in much the same way that too much heat evaporates water in a pot. Yin Qi is linked to water. It cools you down and affects the bodily fluids. A deficiency of Yin Qi in organs is linked to chronic illnesses and it ensures that the organs do not overheat. Just like water, Yin Qi replenishes and cools but an excess is a little like having a waterlogged field.

QI AND THE GAN

After many generations and much trial and error, Jiangan masters eventually discovered that a pole of a certain length, grasped in a particular way, creates a peculiar sensation within the body. It is as though we become 'charged with energy' going through the movements. They also found that there are dramatic health improvements when practising with the Gan which do not manifest when the same movements are made with empty hands. They therefore formulated the concept that the Gan somehow helps Qi cultivation. With further observation and experimentation they declared the following:

- When the Gan is held to the body, it maintains Qi.

- When the Gan moves away or towards the body, it creates Qi.

- When the Gan and body move together, Qi is circulated.

In addition they proposed that the Gan creates a 'pyramid of energy' with the body, the Gan serving as the base of the pyramid.

Pyramids, Triangles and Cones

It is a fascinating suggestion that geometric shapes can somehow affect the human body. The pyramid created in Jiangan is essentially a triangle; the angle is calculated from where the hands grip the Gan (usually at the ends) to the tip of the triangle. This tip is called the vertex (Figures V and VI). The location of the vertex in the human body is based on traditional Chinese medicine which, like Yoga, has identified certain points in the human body where energy gathers or can be directed. But before I deal with these points, there is one more important factor relating to the shape formed by the Gan. Rotating a pyramid or triangle around an axis – which we do when practising Jiangan – creates a cone shape which has long been associated with mysterious esoteric power. Conical (cone-shaped) hats are pointy headgear given to schoolchildren to wear as punishment for misbehaviour or stupidity. The origin of the dunce cap goes back to a group of thirteenth-century esoteric philosophers led by John Duns Scotus of Scotland, who believed that the shape enhanced knowledge by drawing in energy from the 'point' or vertex. The belief that wearing conical hats would funnel learning down to the wearer was reflected by the term 'dunce' being used for slow learners who had to wear the headgear. Similar caps were used in the tribunals of the Spanish Inquisition for questioning heretics. Historically, many types of esoteric practices have used the cone shape to 'work with energy'; witches

36

and wizards are depicted wearing such hats and magicians create a 'Cone of Power' built around a circular base (the 'magic circle') where energy spirals up into a vertex focused on whatever needs to be worked on, using visualisation.

Whether the vertices of cones, triangles or pyramids have 'power' is open to debate, but the terminology of physics throws an interesting light on the matter. A vertex is described as a point where particles collide and interact and 'vertex function' is when a photon and electron interact. One thing is clear: a vertex is a meeting place of two forces.

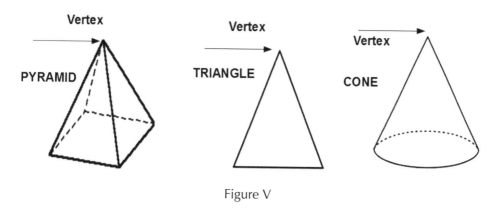

Figure V

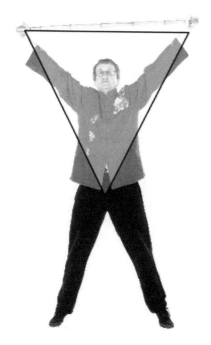
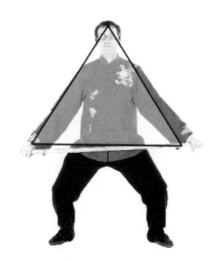

Figure VI

The Yin and Yang Polarities

When practising Jiangan, Qi is focused by the 'pyramid' (the combined shape of the body and the Gan) and accumulates at a tip or vertex corresponding to the body's two main Yin and Yang centres, which are located at the base of the spine and the crown of the head respectively. These two points, in traditional Chinese medicine, are linked via meridian channels. Unlike the 12 'standard' meridian channels that are associated with specific internal organs and worked on by acupuncture and specialist Qigong, these two points are the focuses of the 'Eight Extraordinary Channels' which serve as reservoirs that keep the 12 standard meridian channels supplied with Qi. When meridians are free of obstruction, generative force flows freely, vital breath circulates with no restriction and the system forms a complete circuit. These Eight Extraordinary Channels are *pathways of energy* and are thought to develop before any other energy pathway in the human body. They are a sort of genetic imprint of our entire being and operate on a deep level and transform 'Jing' or Essence into Qi and blood, which in turn supports the 'Shen' or Spirit. It is thought that at conception of humans, the two most important channels, the 'Du Mai' and 'Ren Mai', are created first.

DU MAI CHANNEL AND THE BAIHUI POINT

First the split of the zygote (cell created from an egg and sperm) creates a central axis in the body; at the rear, the 'Du Mai' or 'Governing Channel', which controls all the Yang channels in the body, is formed. When Dr Cheng instructed Bruce Johnson to move energy from a point at the 'Perineum' under the tail bone to the top of the head, we can say with certainty that this is the route of the 'Du Mai', which runs from the Perineum up the spine to the top of the head. Yang is heat, which rises, so Qi rises up the spine regulating and stimulating meridian points on its upward journey. The Baihui point is situated on the crown of the head and corresponds to the Sahasrara (Crown Chakra) in Yoga and is the point at which all the body's Yang energy converges in the Du Mai channel.

Baihui, being Yang in nature, is the link to Heavenly Qi and so 'raising' this point has many health benefits such as improving circulation to the brain and straightening the spine. The modern sedentary lifestyle of sitting constantly at computers or lounging on sofas causes a pathologically curved spine, which manifests as stiffness, back pain, headaches, and other health problems. By raising the crown of your head, you can decompress your spinal vertebrae, strengthen your back, and improve your posture and health. This straightened spine will improve your balance. In most Jiangan exercises we are aware of raising this point. It is essential to tuck in the chin. From an average person's perspective, the Baihui is located towards the back of the head and so lifting it requires a slight forward rotation that brings the chin down and inwards. The Jiangan exercises 'Peeling the Octopus' and 'Twisting the Snake' train you to bring your head into the correct position because the Gan passes behind the back of the head and neck and so requires the head to rotate forwards slightly bringing the spine into correct alignment and also aligning the Baihui with the 'Huiyin' (see below).

REN MAI CHANNEL AND THE HUIYIN POINT

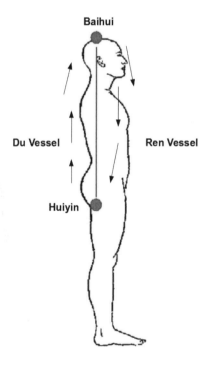

Baihui

Du Vessel

Ren Vessel

Huiyin

Figure VII

At the front of the body the 'Conception Channel' or Ren Mai is the second to be formed from the split in the zygote. This channel directs all the Yin channels in the body. Yin is water, which flows downward. Qi flows down the front of the body like a waterfall and stimulates centres and meridian points on its downward journey to the Perineum. The Huiyin point is located at the Perineum and is the point at which all the body's Yin energy converges at the base of the Ren Mai Channel. It corresponds to the Muladhara or Root Chakra in Yoga. Because this point is the gate through which Qi from other organs can be either retained or lost, it is called the 'Gate of Life and Death'. Being Yin it is connected to the element Earth and hence corresponds to the physical plane of existence, and is (through the feet) the main link with 'Earth Qi'. The Huiyin point is a deep, dark, hidden and protected place where Yin meets. According to Hatha Yoga, the energy of the Muladhara chakra ascends through the centre of the spinal column until it reaches the crown of the head. In Yoga, energy stored at the base of the spine is depicted as a sleeping dragon (in ordinary humans who have not learnt how to develop the energy). This rising energy is associated with life energy, the will, the self, which rises to the crown of the head where Yin mixes with Yang. Similarly, in Daoist Yoga, Qi is directed to the Huiyin and then up the Governing Vessel to the Baihui – albeit by a more complex method. We can now understand why Dr Cheng spoke of energy rising from the base of the spine to the top of the head. Figure VII shows both the general course of the Du Mai and Ren Mai Vessels and the Baihui and Huiyin points.

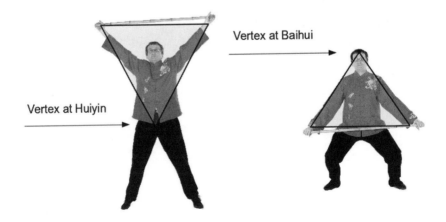

Figure VIII

These two points – the Du Mai Channel's Baihui and the Ren Mai Channel's Huiyin – serve as the body's polarities for Yin and Yang energy. Jiangan exercises become a focus for healing energy channelled through these two points, which are the Yin and Yang Gateways of the body. In Jiangan we are essentially aligning these points with the vertex of the triangle we create (Figure VIII). This simplifies the Chinese energy system into its most basic Yin/Yang control centres and also links with Yoga's Chakra principles.

Jiangan provides Yin-Yang balance through focus on these two points.

ANCIENT GEOMETRY AND THE TWO POLARITIES OF THE HUMAN BODY

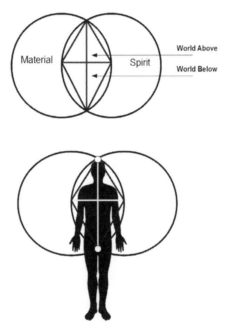

Figure IX

The Baihui and Huiyin points have an importance beyond Chinese internal medicine and the Indian Chakra system. In terms of the human body and how shapes affect it, let us take a look at the origin of basic shapes created by the 'sacred geometry' that runs through many great civilisations. First we have the circle that represents spirit and the universal. In ancient Chinese philosophy, heaven is round and so are the natural forms in nature (planets and birds' nests for example). The square represents matter, rationality and human nature and implies human construction. In Chinese philosophy, the earth is square. The squared circle is a fusion of opposites; temples and religious places throughout the world are founded on squared circle constructions.

The birth of the triangle occurs when two circles are drawn with their centres on the circumference of the other; the overlap creates the 'Vesica Piscis' (Piscine Vessel). The right hand circle represents the spirit realm, which penetrates the material world of the left circle. In a rhombus created in the overlapping area, two equilateral triangles are formed, representing the world above and the world below. The longer axis of the Vesica Piscis (within the two triangles) is positive and the shorter is negative.

The vertices of the upper and lower triangles correspond to the Baihui and Huiyin points of the human body.

The relationship between the Piscean Vessel and the Baihui-Huiyin points in the body has not, to my knowledge, been explored before in any philosophy – certainly not in relation to the Indian-Chinese energy systems. But when the human shape is superimposed on the Piscean Vessel, we can clearly see that the Baihui and Huiyin points align themselves so that the vertex of the upper triangle corresponds to Yang/Heaven and the vertex of the lower triangle corresponds to Yin/Earth. This symbol represents the points at which the Yang and Yin energies in both humans and the universe converge (Figure IX).

Getting Qi into the Body

Once we understand that the vertex of the pyramid/triangle/cone is focused on the Baihui and Huiyin points, the question arises, how do we attract Qi into the body in the first place? In Jiangan as we hold the Gan, we maintain sensitivity to receiving and transmitting energy mainly through the hands. In the wide grip with the hands forming a fist, the palm and fingers should be in contact with the Gan (Figure X). This allows us to focus on feeling the Qi flow into the Gan at the point where our hands grasp it. Qi is drawn into the ends of the Gan and along its length, through the palms and fingers, up the arms and through the body (see Figure XI). There are two acupuncture points on fingers which must be noted here, because they undoubtedly take an active part in receiving and distributing Qi around the body (see Figure XII):

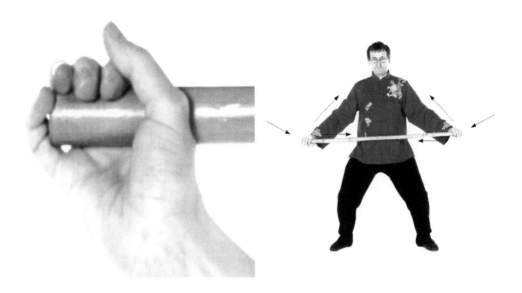

Figure X   Figure XI

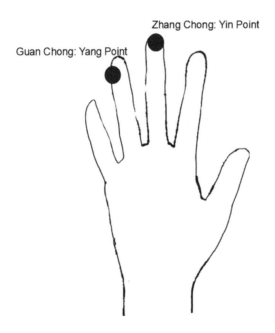

Figure XII

- The Zhang Chong point at the end of the middle finger, which is part of the 'Pericardium Organ' or Xin Bao, a Yin point.

- The Guan Chong point at the end of the fourth or ring finger, which is part of the 'Triple Burner Organ' or San Jiao, a Yang point.

When Qi travels up the arms (and along the Gan to the other hand and arm – the theory is that the Qi will not escape but recirculate around the body), it enters the upper body where the paired Triple Burner (Yang) and Pericardium (Yin) organs meet, and then sinks to the lower body, circulating through all the major internal organs.

THE DAN TIAN

The Dan Tian, one of the most important energy focus points in traditional Chinese medicine, broadly corresponds to the chakra in Yoga. These are located in different parts of the body and the most important for Chinese internal systems is the Dan Tian located in the abdomen. This is about two inches below the navel and two inches behind – the location of the body's centre of gravity. This point is equivalent to the Manipura or navel chakra in Yoga. In Daoist Alchemy the Dan Tian is the focus of energy before it is lowered to the base of the spine and lifted to the top of the head. The Jiangan practitioner may want to focus on energy in the navel Dan Tian before 'following' it mentally down into the Huiyin, where it will rise up the back of the body to the Baihui point.

MICROCOSMIC ORBIT MEDITATION

The above process is essentially a simplified version of a process from ancient Daoist Alchemy called microcosmic orbit meditation. It is primarily a form of sitting meditation that does not involve exercise. Starting at the midline, the practitioner imagines Qi rising up the spine, over the head to the face then down to the chest and belly, down under the genitals, then back up the spine to continue this orbit over and over again. First the practitioner generates Qi in his or her navel Dan Tian, then opens the various energy centres along the microcosmic orbit route where the Qi must pass (Figure VII shows the general orbit). Unblocking these energy centres is a process sometimes called

'Kai Men' or 'Opening the Doors'. Daoist Yoga, which is related to Jiangan, is also known as Kai Men. Jiangan vastly simplifies the microcosmic orbit but similarly achieves the opening of the various doors along the energy centres. The major advantage of Jiangan is that the body receives additional exercise as it performs the orbit.

EGYPTIAN RODS

There is a remarkable parallel between traditional Chinese medicine, Yoga and certain practices of ancient Egypt that is relevant to Jiangan. A method of strengthening 'energy flows' within the human body was devised involving two rods, one of which was clutched in each hand. The idea was to create an electrical conduit, gather it in the spinal fluid, then harmonise the two main energy streams which corresponded to the concepts of 'Yin' and 'Yang'. The rods were designed for use by the Pharaohs. The Yang rod was held in the right hand and represented the god Horus, who symbolises the flow of Yang energy. The Yin rod was held in the left hand and represented the goddess Hathor, who symbolises the female principle and the flow of Yin energy. The use of these rods was said to have had a beneficial effect on the Pharaoh's health. The (Sun/Yang) rod for the right hand was made from copper, reinforced by gold, and the (Moon/Yin) rod for the left hand was made from zinc and reinforced by silver.

The Egyptians, like the Buddhists, regarded the right hand as 'Yang' and left hand 'Yin' but some Daoist Alchemical sources have the right hand as Yin and left hand Yang. Since Jiangan is influenced by Daoist Yoga, the right hand can be taken as Yin and the left as Yang. So Qi can be visualised entering the ends of the Gan; at the right (Yin) side travelling up the arm through the palm or moving along the Gan and up the left arm; while Qi enters the left (Yang) end of the Gan and up the left arm. The Qi, thus entering the body on both sides of the Gan, proceeds into the body and down to the navel Dan Tian, sinking to the Huiyin then up the spine to the Baihui on top of the head. The circulation of Qi is certainly something to ponder during practice but it is not necessary to associate a particular hand with Yin or Yang, nor even to visualise the flow of Qi along the Gan in any particular direction. It is enough that we are sensitive to the energy entering though the fingers that are attached lightly to the Gan; we may, if we are especially sensitive, feel Qi

45

travelling up the arms, into the body and down into the Dan Tian, and then to the base of the spine where it travels up to the top of the head. A specific healing methodology – if there was one in Jiangan – may have been lost in the mists of time, but general health and well-being certainly result from regular Jiangan practice.

ENERGY ACTIVATION IN JIANGAN

The microcosmic orbit is incorporated in Jiangan using pyramid energy. The basic theory is that when we lower the Gan horizontally, the pyramid creates a vertex in the Baihui point on the top of the head; when the Gan is raised horizontally the pyramid creates a vertex in the Huiyin point in the Perineum (Figure VIII). We can, for example, focus our thoughts and meditate on heat or fire rising at the rear of the body (up the spine, the Yang path) as Qi rises. But Qi must also sink, and although this is not specifically mentioned in Johnson's text, it can be logically inferred. Just as throwing a ball requires a backward motion of the arm, energy must first sink before it rises. So to get this balance there must also be a Yin awareness of Qi sinking, perhaps as cooling water flowing down the front of the body to the Huiyin point. Combined with breathing and constant movement between Yin and Yang extremes, this microcosmic orbit meditation is a potent yet simple affirmation of ancient Chinese philosophy.

YIN-YANG AND RESISTANCE

The Yin-Yang principle is at the heart of Jiangan's body mechanics. In most exercises, parts of the body are immobile (Yin) while other parts move (Yang). This creates the gentle resistance which stretches and massages muscles and massages internal organs.

5

Methodology

BREATHING: ONE BREATH TO RULE THEM ALL

Breathing is one of our most vital functions because it brings oxygen to the blood and the brain. Breathing exercises have been shown to help control respiratory problems as well as psychological conditions like anxiety, panic attacks, phobias and depression. The regular practice of breathing exercises can also be energising, relaxing and improve concentration. There are many thousands of types of breathing exercises. In Yoga there are methods with such descriptive names as 'Victorious Breath', 'Humming Bee', 'Cooling Breath', 'Alternate Nostril Breathing', 'Shining Skull' and 'Bellows Breath. In Qigong some of the many breathing techniques include 'Pre-birth' or 'Reverse Breathing' and 'Tortoise Breathing'. Breathing is also a fundamental element of Jiangan. The movements follow the breathing and if there is no breathing, there is no movement and no exercise. So we should not think of Jiangan as exercise with breathing but breathing with exercise.

Jiangan uses only *one* type of breathing – natural deep breathing, also called diaphragmatic breathing, which involves expanding the diaphragm when inhaling and contracting it when exhaling. This type of breathing can be observed in sleeping animals and babies; their stomachs expand and contract as they breathe. By contrast, many humans – especially elderly people – practise 'shallow breathing' where the chest expands and contracts. Diaphragmatic breathing is essentially breathing from the navel Dan Tian region where Qi is brought during exercise to be distributed throughout the body. This type of deep diaphragmatic breathing has many beneficial and healing qualities such as:

- Relaxing the muscles surrounding the small blood vessels and allowing the blood to flow more easily.

- Allowing alpha blockers to block receptors in arteries and smooth muscles.

- Relaxing blood vessels, leading to an increase in blood flow and lowering pressure to control hypertension.

- Enhancing urinary flow in the urinary tract and reducing the risk and symptoms of an enlarged prostate.

- Releasing endorphins that help relieve symptoms of premenstrual syndrome.

Diaphragmatic breathing is also called 'Yang' breath because the exhalation (Yang) is longer than the inhalation (Yin). This is important because complete exhalation clears 'stale air' that can cause many ills (stale air is carbon dioxide, wastes and toxins that accumulate in the lungs). Many types of meditation employ the ratio of 1:2 or 1:3 inhalation-exhalation, and Johnson follows this method in his book. The natural extension of this is to use timing which the body is most attuned to.

Golden Ratio Breathing

Using the Fibonacci numbers for convenience, if we inhale for three seconds we find that we naturally exhale for about five seconds or even up to eight seconds if we are especially meditative. With this three second inhalation ratio, the more experienced may be able to go up to a thirteen second exhalation. This is the body finding its natural rhythm, which is aligned to the Golden Ratio (Figure XIII). Listening to someone sleeping peacefully you will hear the pattern where the exhalation lasts longer than the inhalation. This timing has been used in various cartoons for comic effect for snoring; the exhalation 'whistle' is longer than the snore in general proportion to the Golden Ratio. The presence of the Golden Ratio in natural relaxed breathing indicates the relationship between the amount of oxygen needed in the blood and the amount of carbon dioxide needed to be sent out, and suggests that Golden Ratio breathing may be one of the great secrets of health.

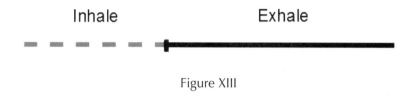

Figure XIII

Try a little exercise. Inhale through your nose for three seconds then immediately exhale through your mouth (pursed 'O' shaped lips making a slight whistling sound) for five seconds. Repeat a few times. This should sound and feel familiar because you are using the basic breathing pattern you employ when you are sleeping and *all of us employ this naturally in the moments before we fall asleep.* This is the time when we start to breathe deeply from the diaphragm. Using this, and only this, type of breathing during Jiangan exercises trains the body to breathe deeply and correctly. While the many specialist breathing methods employed by Yoga and Qigong have specific beneficial effects, Golden Ratio deep diaphragmatic breathing is the simplest and most effective natural method to employ during a daily exercise regime.

POSTURE AND BREATHING

The 'wide grip' (holding the Gan at the ends) opens the chest and strongly encourages correct posture for efficient breathing. The deep breathing resulting from this posture may be more effective than other types of breathing exercises because it 'turbo-charges' the breathing process.

BREATHING METHOD

Inhalation through the nose and exhalation through the mouth is the norm in Jiangan, but with exercises demanding a little more effort, the double inhalation method is employed. Here we inhale through the nose and mouth simultaneously but still exhale though the mouth as normal. This method will become second nature once you have discovered when you need to employ it and it will vastly enhance the benefits of the exercises.

GRADUATED STAGES

If one characteristic sets Jiangan apart from all other exercises, it is the graduated stages methodology. Here is the basic method. Imagine that an exercise requires that you bend to touch your toes. Most systems would perform this in one movement, then either hold the posture for a set number of seconds or repeat it a set number of times. If breathing also accompanies the exercise, usually there is only one 'breathing cycle' employed (i.e. exhale while bending and inhale while returning upright). To get the benefit of, say, ten breathing cycles you would have to repeat the whole exercise ten times. In Jiangan this imaginary toe-touching exercise would be broken up into five stages, each going a little further towards the 'goal' of touching the toes – but significantly, each stage has its own breathing cycle.

This has many advantages. First the practitioner gradually prepares his or her muscles for the stretch and bend. It also ensures that muscles get more oxygen and that there is more breathing benefit with less stress on the body. Graduated stages also make it easier for people of varying physical abilities to perform exercises because they can set smaller targets for themselves. Each stage becomes a 'micro exercise' within itself. After each stage the practitioner returns to the beginning stage before moving to the next, until the body's comfortable limit is reached. Fit and healthy people should aim to perform the final stage of each exercise as demonstrated in this book. But Jiangan is very adaptable and makes allowances for individual ability. Infirm and elderly people and those out of condition can use what I call the 'Inch-by-Inch' method, which is described in Chapter 8. Even though there are many people who will not be able to progress very far, they are still performing Jiangan. There is, however, no reason why the average able-bodied person cannot progress to the final positions shown in this book. But no matter how fit or healthy you are, you must *not* skip the five stages. The graduated stages method not only guards against strains and injury but also gives Jiangan its unique potency. Remember, do not rush through the exercises. They are not physical but internal.

Johnson linked the five stages to the Five Chinese Elements in 'mutual creation' order: earth creates metal, metal creates water, water creates wood, wood creates fire. The exercises start with 'Yin' and end with 'Yang' so making seven actual stages in all (Figure XIV). It is not necessary to link the stages to the elements but meditation on them has many advantages, including the following:

- Enhancing the experience.

- Ensuring that the postures are performed correctly and not rushed.

- Making it easier to remember the points where the Gan must reach for each stage.

- The union of the Five Elements produces the elixir of immortality!

Final Stage	Yang	阳
Stage 5	Fire	火
Stage 4	Wood	木
Stage 3	Water	水
Stage 2	Metal	金
Stage 1	Earth	土
Beginning Stage	Yin	阴

Figure XIV

Figure XV shows some of the 'Correspondences' of the Five Elements in Chinese philosophy and it is beneficial to employ meditations and visualisations while performing the graduated stages.

Stage	Element	Organs	Colour	Voice	Flavour	Climate
Beginning Yin						
1	Earth	Stomach/Spleen	Yellow	Singing	Sweet	Humidity
2	Metal	Lungs/Large Intestine	White	Crying	Hot	Dryness
3	Water	Bladder/Kidneys	Black	Groaning	Salty	Cold
4	Wood	Liver/Gallbladder	Green	Shouting	Sour	Wind
5	Fire	Heart/Small Intestine	Red	Laughing	Bitter	Hot
Final Yang						

Figure XV

SAFETY

There is no greater consideration for an exercise than safety, especially exercises for ordinary people who are not in the best physical shape. Health and safety specialists these days tell us that when lifting heavy objects, we should always bend our knees and keep the back straight to avoid risk of injury. This methodology has not spring up from nowhere but was the result of experience; it is the *only* way that 'works', and so logically the same methodology must also be true for any person in the ancient world who wanted to lift heavy objects, and will remain a truth for future generations. In most human endeavours an optimum method or technique is developed and it is invariably discovered after many years of experiment, trial and error. The methodology of Jiangan is probably the safest ever devised because the masters developed exercises that were not only beneficial but also safe to practise each day, every day of a person's life.

How did the masters know what was safe and what was not? How did they know which postures, positions and movements had positive effects on the body and which had negative effects? Not by guesswork, religious dogma or intellectual theory, but simply by observation, experimentation, trial and error over centuries. Time may be a great healer but it is a much better teacher. All important human activities, including art, hunting, building, toolmaking and farming, have benefited from the refinement of techniques made by successive generations. Jiangan masters, like all artisans, rejected what was bad or ineffective and kept what was good and what worked. This approach resulted in vastly superior and safer exercises than the 'traditional' ones taught in schools, colleges and military establishments in the West, many of which have sprung up from intellectual or academic ideas rather than long experience. This is because people in the West have been practising and studying exercise seriously for only a few decades, whereas people in the East have thousands of years' experience.

Jiangan is Good for the Knees

The knee is more of a weight-transferring joint than a weight-bearing joint. Although the body's entire weight is frequently placed all on one leg, this is usually very briefly when walking or climbing, and the knee transfers weight across the body. Exercises must play to the knees' strengths and avoid their weaknesses. Traditional lunges put all the body's weight onto one leg for longer, more intense periods which puts undue pressure on the knee joint. Two Jiangan exercises ('Horse Stance on a Tightrope' and 'The Tiger Springs') are brilliantly devised so that the knees are spared excess pressure. This is because weight is evenly distributed on both legs and in the latter exercise the feet are also angled out so that the pressure is taken off the knees completely. This methodology is evidence of many years' experience of trial and error of different methods until the safest and most efficient one was found. Fitness trainers in the West have only recently begun to use similar methodology as Jiangan's 'The Tiger Springs' in which the practitioner steps forwards with one foot but actually distributes the weight equally, so that the knees are not under undue pressure.

However, coming from a Taiji background, some methods of Jiangan were against my instincts. Out of the 17 Exercises Routine, three exercises ('Bowing', 'Greeting the Traveller' and 'Search for the Hatchet') require locked knees in a standing position. With most conventional exercises involving locked knees, the body extends to the extreme position in one energetic movement and either holds that position or repeats the entire movement over and over in a jerky manner. But Jiangan employs the graduated stages methodology and so, although our knees are locked, we move gradually into the exercise in small, slow and gentle movements and only go as far as we feel comfortable. In addition we do not stay in the end position much longer than a change of breath. Locking knees in these particular exercises allows you to stand without using the quadriceps to hold the legs in a straight position, which is an energy-efficient mechanism that avoids muscular contraction. It is also a methodology to ensure that the body is held in a secure, stable and consistent posture for the duration of the exercise. Because locked knees prevent individuals from 'going awry', the technique can be used to maintain consistency and is a very scientific approach that will be invaluable in future medical research. Therefore, using the graduated stages protects the joints, muscles and tendons and ensures that the gradual progression to the individual's natural Yang position is beneficial and safe. I also suspect that locking the knees in these three exercises contributes to strengthening the whole knee region. I have had chronic soreness in my left knee for most of my life but after practising Jiangan daily for over a year, the problem disappeared and has never returned. In fact both knees have strengthened considerably. So although avoiding locking knees is a good general rule for most types of exercise, it is not intrinsically bad otherwise my knee would have got worse. And, of course, the masters over the centuries would have noticed ill effects from locking knees in these three exercises, especially as they took great pains to make the other exercises in the system safe. It is good methodology that steers us away from injury. I am also convinced that the sequence and holistic method of the entire 17 Exercises Routine plays a huge role in avoiding injury and improving the general condition of the knees. Directly after exercises requiring locked knees comes the safe squat and lunge. So all the muscle groups that support the knee and control knee movement and stability – particularly the quadriceps and the hamstrings – are gently stretched and strengthened in turn and in the most beneficial sequence.

Having practised Taiji for over 30 years, the major reason I adopted Jiangan as a daily exercise was that it is kinder on my knees. After a round of Taiji my naturally weak left knee sometimes feels hot and sore (though this happens less now that my knees have been strengthened with Jiangan) but after practising Jiangan there is no problem at all. So is Taiji good for the knees? That is like asking whether strenuous exercise is good for the heart. It depends on the state of the individual's heart to begin with: while strenuous exercise can strengthen the heart, people with pre-existing heart conditions will have problems. It is the same with Taiji and knees. Healthy fit people with no knee problems will have no difficulty in performing Taiji as they shift their weight constantly from one leg to the other so that about 70 per cent is placed on each leg in turn (one of the most distinctive features of Taiji). But this methodology does put quite a bit of pressure on the knee. When I started learning many years ago, I was taught the correct method of securing 'safe' knees such as ensuring the joint is in alignment and that the knee does not extend beyond the toes. But after many years of practising 'correctly', trying different theories and styles and experimenting with postures and alignment, my left knee was still habitually prone to hot soreness after a round of Taiji practice. Clearly, people with inherent weaknesses in their knees can perform Taiji comfortably only if the methodology is amended. So we must say that as a complete health exercise, Taiji is a 'work in progress' and further evolution is needed if it is to develop as a comprehensive health practice.

Jiangan is Good for the Back

There are three exercises in Jiangan that involve bending forwards in standing position (again, 'Bowing', 'Greeting the Traveller' and 'Search for the Hatchet'). In this respect they are similar to many Yoga and Daoist Yoga exercises. In recent years some Western exercise instructors have questioned whether forward bending from a standing position puts injurious pressure on the discs. They are primarily reacting to the type of exercise that requires a forward bend to the extreme position in one go, often with jerky or bouncing movements or at speed. This has led some fitness instructors to advise avoidance of all bending forward exercises under any circumstances. Some Yoga teachers have even been encouraged to attend 're-education seminars' to change the methodology of Yoga to avoid forward bending completely. The West, it seems, likes to take the chauvinistic attitude of 'starting everything again' as if the thousands of years of Indian and Chinese culture and experience in exercise never happened!

It should be noted that Eastern health arts are not superstitions or fads (like foot-binding). The ancient methods of improving the body have been passed down, generation-to-generation, teacher-to-student, and many very elderly practitioners of Yoga and Qigong can be found today who have been performing forward bends all their lives, not only without injury but also with increased health and strength of the back. One must ask whether these legions of dedicated practitioners failed to notice that their profoundly worked out postures were harmful to certain parts of the body?

We must conclude that Indian and Chinese observations and experiences are valid and that the academic theories that condemn them are flawed and without basis in experience. Eastern methods of exercise are very different from Western exercises not only because of the philosophical and religious aspects but simply because these ancient civilisations have devised the best ways to exercise mind, body and spirit safely and constructively. Jiangan is a perfect example; risk associated with forward bending is negligible largely because the graduated stages methodology protects the back and the joints and ensures that we never strain ourselves or traumatise any part of the body. But if you want to be even more cautious, you can perform bends well within your own comfort zone, which may mean bending for only a few inches in some circumstances. Using the safe methodology, you will notice that your back will respond favourably to the exercises and get stronger.

As with all exercises, if you have a specific medical complaint you are advised to consult your doctor before taking up Jiangan. Johnson encouraged readers doubtful of the art to take his book along to a doctor and I can only echo this sentiment. By all means show this book to your doctor, physiotherapist or sports trainer. There are, of course, some people who are unable to do some of the exercises in this book and many people will not be able to go into the final positions of many postures. Therefore individuals must go only as far as they are able to, and create their own Yang position. Sometimes there will have to be considerable adaptation – but do not change the basic shape of the posture or the breathing method. Adaptation means being aware of how far to proceed in each exercise towards your own final Yang stage. Accordingly, each exercise has adaptation notes for those unable to proceed to the ideal Yang positions.

Safe Stretching

Undoubtedly resulting from its roots in animal observation, stretching is an important element of Jiangan. Stretching is deliberate lengthening of muscles and is an excellent way to become more flexible, increase joint mobility, prevent training injuries, improve circulation and posture, and relieve muscle stress. Stretching also maintains the pliability of muscles thus avoiding injuries while taking part in sport. It increases range of motion and flexibility and helps remove waste products from the blood. It also reduces the chances of muscle soreness after exercise because stiff, less flexible muscles receive more muscle fibre damage in training which results in loss of muscle strength. In Jiangan we stretch by slowly and gently relaxing the muscles using the graduated stages – the safest way to stretch. We first work the back, shoulders, arms and neck, then the legs and finally the muscles in the centre of the body. When one muscle group is exercised, we then exercise the opposite or related muscle group, which is the most efficient method.

SPEED, TIMING AND REPETITIONS

Because the pace of the exercises is slow and regulated by deep breathing, the body finds its own rhythm. If you go too fast you will be performing a 'physical' exercise and your muscles will be tense, making it difficult to stretch safely. It is also difficult to breathe deeply if you move too fast. Be relaxed and move at a gentle pace and the circulation in your cardiovascular system will improve without the shocks and trauma to the joints, muscles and internal organs that occur with more robust exercises.

Most exercise systems require the practitioner to hold a position for a certain length of time or repeat it a certain number of times. Usually there is no logical reason for these timings. Breathing is the foundation of movement in Jiangan. The body is not generally 'held' in the Yang stage of an exercise for longer than a change of breath and only in a few exercises is there an instruction to hold the last repetition for a few seconds or so. This is a guideline, not a hard-and-fast rule. Jiangan's philosophy on timing and repetition can be encapsulated in the Chinese adage, 'A journey of a thousand miles begins with a single step.' In other words a little effort is all you need to make progress. Once you have completed the graduated stages and got to your Yang stage, the number of repetitions is left up to you. You simply repeat the Yin to Yang sequence as many times as you feel you are able. Some people may want to do only one repetition and with others just getting to the Yang stage is enough. As the most important element is the *journey* to the Yang stage, benefit has already been obtained performing the graduated stages.

Jiangan is the only exercise system which has this methodology. In addition, although we are instructed to repeat two of the exercises a minimum number of times, this is again only a recommendation to get the best out of the postures. I cannot stress strongly enough that if you find a particular exercise difficult, perform fewer repetitions or advance more slowly, but *do not* change the structure of the exercises themselves or miss any of them out.

GRIP

As we grasp the Gan we make a light 'fist' using the sort of grip used to hold the Taiji sword. It is also the grip a baby uses to grasp a finger – firm but not aggressive or too tight. Although the baby does not use force or tension, it is quite difficult to pull your finger away. Without knowing it, babies use true Qi energy. So hold the Gan firmly but not tightly. If you are not sure of the correct pressure to use, repeated practice will eventually reveal the balanced grip – or, rather, refamiliarise yourself with the grip of your infancy. As mentioned in Chapter 4, it is important for 'Qi gathering' to grasp the Gan so that as much of the palm and fingers are in contact with it as possible.

6

Questions and Answers

Q: *Is Jiangan a martial art?*

A: No. Jiangan is a daily health maintenance exercise. Martial arts schools can use the system for combined warm-ups, stretching and breathing exercises, but Jiangan has a non-martial methodology and philosophy.

Q: *How often should I practise?*

A: Preferably you should practise every day. I frequently practise twice a day: once in the morning and once in the evening, and sometimes put in a light session at lunchtime (only proceeding to one or two stages of each exercise).

Q: *What time of day is best to practise?*

A: Any time of day that suits you, but you should leave about an hour after meals and an hour or so after you wake up in the morning. It is also best not to exercise too late at night because you may be too alert to sleep.

Q: *How long does it take to perform the 17 Exercises Routine?*

A: The length of time varies according to the individual and how many Yin to Yang repetitions he or she performs. To perform the exercises correctly you should allow at least 20 minutes, but 30 minutes or over is not unusual. If you have extreme time constraints it is possible to perform the entire routine in about 10 or 15 minutes but only by omitting all but the first one or two stages of each exercise. Even though people do not have much spare time in the modern world, you should not be judging an exercise routine on the length of time it takes to perform. Nobody would suggest that a convenience meal 'ready in two minutes' is more nourishing than a carefully prepared meal, yet this logic is increasingly used to sell exercises to time-conscious consumers in the modern world.

Q: *How much room do I need?*
A: You only really need space to hold the Gan in the various positions of each exercise. You could get through a routine in a space six foot square.

Q: *What clothing should I wear?*
A: Anything that is comfortable but do not wear anything too loose or flowing in case it gets in the way of the Gan.

Q: *What footwear should I use and can I perform Jiangan in my bare feet?*
A: One of the most noticeable differences between Indian and Chinese methods of exercises is that the Chinese tend to wear shoes (certainly with Qigong and Taiji) whereas Yoga practitioners practise in bare feet. While there is no definite instruction from Dr Cheng one way or the other, it is both in keeping with Chinese tradition and also a result of personal experience that I advise wearing flat comfortable shoes when performing Jiangan. I have tried practising in bare feet but found that footwear makes the postures more secure and easier to hold.

Q: *Doesn't Yoga also achieve external body-shaping effects such as toning muscles and aiding weight loss?*
A: Yoga is an excellent and profound health system with implications far beyond mere physical well-being. However, it is complex, with hundreds of different exercises and breathing systems. Unlike Jiangan, it did not evolve one single simple methodology aimed at providing a daily exercise suitable for everyone. In recent years with the popularity of Yoga, many

simplified exercises have been devised for that purpose but these routines are not as 'tried and tested' as Jiangan, which has been doing this specific task for much longer.

Q: *I have seen many styles of sticks and implements used in Taiji and Qigong. Isn't Jiangan simply another of these variants?*

A: There are indeed a range of training implements used in both Qigong and Taiji, such as the 'Taiji ball', 'ruler' and 'bang' (small sticks), to enhance certain aspects of Taiji and Qigong training. The 'Taiji ruler' is an interesting device – a small stick about the size and shape of a rolling pin that is rolled in the palms to 'cultivate Qi'. Despite claims that these implements can be traced back hundreds of years and were practised by certain emperors (a familiar story!), most authorities seem to agree that the 'ruler', 'ball' and 'bang' were most probably developed around the early years of the twentieth century or perhaps even later. This suggested era brings up an interesting fact that although the Chinese martial arts are ancient, the period just after the turn of the twentieth century saw the birth of many forms and weapons routines. It may be significant that these emerged in the wake of the Boxer Rebellion just a few years earlier. Although this historic event was the catalyst for the general surge of interest in internal arts and martial arts in China, there is little evidence that Jiangan came out of the same melting pot. Its body mechanics and methodology are quite foreign to modern Qigong and Taiji. We can say with some confidence that the 'Wand' is the most ancient of Chinese internal health aids.

Q: *I cannot lock my knees. Can I practise with my knees slightly bent?*

A: The main reason for locked knees in the exercises that require this methodology is to stabilise the body and maintain secure and consistent posture. You should make every effort to lock your knees when you perform these exercises but if you are medically unable to, you can slightly bend your knees – but do not bend them too much because this will destabilise your posture and this may eventually cause problems. Remember, the methods of Jiangan were not arrived at by whim but from long years of observation and trial and error.

Q: *Is there a special health diet recommended with Jiangan?*

A: The Imperial family would probably be unwilling to eliminate fine food and wine from their diet and so while many Daoists and Chinese internal artists recommend foods according to how much 'Yin' and 'Yang' they possess (resulting in some remarkably frugal eating habits), there are no such restrictions in Jiangan. Many of these dietary prohibitions are based only on theories rather than practical experience over many centuries, which makes them unreliable. But that does not mean we are free to eat anything we desire. We must try to eradicate as much salt, sugar and saturated fat as we can, and to avoid processed food, eat fresh fruit and vegetables and wholemeal bread and brown rice instead of the refined variety.

Q: *Sports scientists have invented many new efficient exercises systems. Why is an ancient exercise like Jiangan so special?*

A: Who is genius enough to devise the 'perfect' exercise system? Individuals are flawed and imperfect and while a genius can, with a spark of inspiration, make a groundbreaking discovery or come up with a fantastic invention that changes the world, in most matters we must work as a team and there is a limit to individual resourcefulness no matter how talented the individual may be. Individuals and committees frequently create exercise systems but none of them is anything approaching perfect, and most contain one flaw or another that was not envisaged at the time of creation. Humans tend to solve problems not in a 'eureka' revolutionary fashion, but in a gradual, evolutionary way, working as a team, with each new generation making a contribution to a particular subject or problem and carrying on the work of their predecessors to take their subjects to new heights. With the development of exercises, there needs to be a certain gestation period to discover flaws and weaknesses – which might amount to many generations – before potential risks are exposed.

Jiangan has been around for many centuries and examined by countless generations; bugs have been fixed and the exercises improved through trial and error and observation. At some point in the past, the exercises reached a point that no further adjustment was needed in the methodology to make it more effective, safer and beneficial.

Q: *Can I tailor Jiangan to my own body rather than practise the same exercises as everyone else?*

A: With some exercise systems the instructor 'tailors' exercises to individual people. This seems a good idea on first inspection because we are all different and may have different exercise needs. However, every human body is essentially the same on the deepest physiological level. Just as medicine and poison affect everyone and dangerous exercises harm everyone, safe, effective exercises are also safe and effective for everyone no matter what their condition or physical state. Jiangan has already been tailored to the human body in general and no matter what the physical shape or condition of the individual, the exercises are effective. Any special needs are accommodated in the 'adaptations' of each exercise.

Q: *Can Jiangan be used as a conditioner and warm-up for any sport or physical activity?*

A: It can certainly serve as a combined warm-up and stretching exercise for most types of sports. It provides a systematic gradual and gentle exercise. Practitioners of any activity will certainly benefit from Jiangan before a class or game because of its integrated and comprehensive nature.

Q: *It is rather dull practising the same exercises every day. Why can't I perform the exercises in a different order or only do some one day and others on another day?*

A: There are some who promote the idea of 'variety' in daily exercises. The theory is that if we perform the same exercises each day it will result in a dull, boring routine repeated ad-nauseam and that varying exercises keeps them 'interesting'. On the face of it this seems logical because nobody wants to be lumbered with dull boring exercises every day. The strategy of varying daily exercise makes sense for more robust physical routines because the body needs to rest certain areas to avoid strains and injury. But for an internal mind-body exercise that can be practised each day with no ill effects, the idea of variety is based solely on psychology, not the physiological needs of the body. Changing exercises each day is not a methodology derived from experience of ancient masters of the East. If the originators of Jiangan, for example, had evidence that variety was beneficial, they would have employed it rather than the ordered

63

daily sequence in the 17 Exercises Routine. The logic of their thinking is clear: if a sequence performed each day has been found most effective for the body, it is like taking the same medicine each day for your long-standing medical condition. No doctor would encourage patients to take a different medicine each day simply for the sake of 'variety'. In other Chinese disciplines such as Taiji and Qigong, the sequence of forms and routines is not changed on a daily basis to avoid boredom, because they have been constructed with a logical intent based on either martial or medical reasons. The sequence of Jiangan has similarly been logically put together for the benefit of the body's all-round health.

Q: *If Jiangan was passed on through different generations, why is it that different styles have not appeared like most other Chinese internal arts?*

A: This is an excellent question. It is probable that the Jiangan masters had to ensure that it remained secret to prevent it being copied. But the art also had to be practised sufficiently regularly by many knowledgeable people. My own view is that 'quality control' was maintained by regular secret meetings supervised by court officials so that practitioners could submit amendments or report problems. A similar process exists in China today where committees comprised of Qigong and Taiji masters evaluate routines for inclusion in official promotions. This ensures consistency and that there is no deviation from methodology that has been shown to be beneficial. Secrecy in Chinese martial arts is often derided or attributed to negative motives. But a certain level of secrecy is beneficial because it maintains control of an art in its development stages. If we see an art practised by different people in many different ways, it can often indicate that it was 'appropriated' by watching eyes before it was perfected.

Q: *Does Jiangan have origins outside China?*

A: It is impossible to say for certain. But it is possible that it could have had its beginnings in India or even Egypt. It may be significant that many of its postures and philosophy resemble the ancient type of Qigong called 'Daoist Yoga', which is similar to Hatha Yoga. This is an exercise system originating in India that incorporates bodily postures (asanas) and breath control (pranayamas), with the focus on moving energy (or prana) along the spine and through the energy centres of the chakras. Some authorities say that Daoist Yoga, which is sometimes called Chinese Yoga or 'Kai Men' (Opening the Doors), is actually a Chinese version of Hatha Yoga, which has been incorporated into Chinese philosophy. Through Daoist Yoga, Jiangan may contain the essence of Yoga's wisdom. The Egyptian Rods offer a fascinating alternate origin of Jiangan.

7

The 17 Exercises Routine
十七势

There are hundreds of Jiangan exercises but most of them are variations or combinations of the 17 Exercises Routine in this book that were designed to be practised by everyone, irrespective of age and physical condition. But the 17 Exercises Routine comprises a complete and comprehensive workout for body, mind and spirit. They are split into ten standing and seven floor exercises. I must stress again that the routine is devised to be practised in one session in the correct sequence as laid out in this book. You must not deviate from this nor miss out an exercise because you do not like it or because you think it is difficult. If you need to adapt any movements, there is advice on doing so after the description section of each exercise. If you have no time to practise all 17 exercises you could split them and practise the standing exercises in the morning and the floor exercises in the evening, but only if you have no other option. While any practice is better than none, make every effort to practise all 17 exercises in one go. If time is a factor it is better to reduce the number of stages performed or the number of repetitions and do the entire routine rather than repeat your favourite exercises and miss out the others. If in doubt about an exercise always err on the side of caution and perform it well within your limits.

A little practice each day is much better than an hour's intense practice a few times a week.

Standing Exercises

1 Stretching the Crane 舒展鹤

This first exercise is the only one performed without the Gan. It is a supreme warm-up for almost any activity and also a complete Qigong exercise that can be practised on its own. There are only two stages.

STAGE 1

Stand straight in a wide stance. Inhale deeply as you rise onto your toes while lifting your arms and stretching them back and out to your sides. At the same time tilt your head back and arch your back slightly. Stretch your arms back behind your body as far as you are able (Figure 1.1).

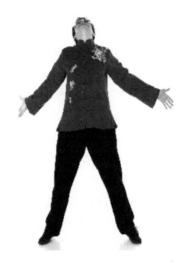

Figure 1.1

STAGE 2

Exhale completely as you come down from your toes and plant both feet on the ground. At the same time bring your arms to the front of your body, placing palms together as if you are praying, and bend over, knees slightly bent, swinging your hands down between your legs (Figure 1.2). It is recommended that you repeat this at least ten times. Figure 1.3 shows the sequence.

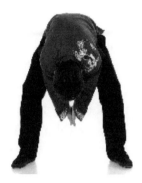

Figure 1.2

Yin-Yang Energy Activation

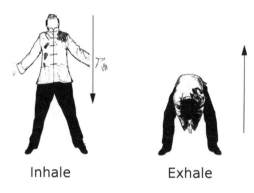

Inhale	Exhale
Yin position: feel cooling water flowing down the front of the body to the Huiyin point at the base of the spine	Yang position: feel fire rising up the spine to the Baihui point at the top of the head

Figure 1.3

ADAPTATION

If you find it hard to stand on your toes, move your weight to the front of your feet as you move into Stage 1. You may eventually be able to raise your heels off the ground in this position. Do not miss this posture just because you have trouble standing on your toes to make the 'perfect' posture or you will miss the great benefits of this exercise.

Notes

This is the exercise that lets you get the feel of the method used in the entire routine (you are learning to move your body to coordinate each inhalation and exhalation). Your speed is controlled by your breathing. The purpose of this exercise is to get the blood to move more efficiently through the body and stimulate muscles. Breathe calmly and not too quickly. As you feel your back, arms and shoulders stretch when you rise onto your toes, you will feel invigorated. Do not become discouraged if you lose your balance. Perseverance will improve your balance and pay dividends when your body gets used to this unusual movement. The strength of this exercise is in its simplicity. There are no complex patterns to learn and the coordination is 'natural' and quickly becomes intuitive. If you want more out of this exercise, imagine that your open palms are gathering 'Heavenly Qi' as you stretch up and back, then as your palms come together between your legs imagine you are focusing the Qi and moving it up your arms and into your body.

2 Sunrise and Sunset 日出日落

BEGINNING STAGE YIN 阴

Grasp the Gan in a wide grip; this is the most frequently used grip in the system. The hands are placed at each end of the Gan with the little finger resting on the ends or in the hollow if using bamboo (Figure 2.1). This ensures that the hands do not slip or slide and maintains the correct width. Stand with feet wide apart, the Gan held up horizontally above your head in line with your nose. Your back should be straight but slightly arched backwards. Do not lean forwards. Inhale deeply as you rise up on your toes and stretch the Gan up as high as you can, keeping it horizontal and in a straight line above the nose (Figure 2.2). Each stage continues from the previous one without pause unless mentioned in the description.

STAGE 1 EARTH 土

Exhale completely as you bring the Gan down from the beginning position, close to your face, to your throat, at the same time coming down from your toes and keeping your back straight (Figure 2.3). Then inhale deeply as you lift the Gan back up to the beginning stage, again rising onto your toes and stretching the body as you lift the Gan as high as you can.

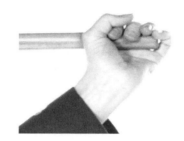

Figure 2.1

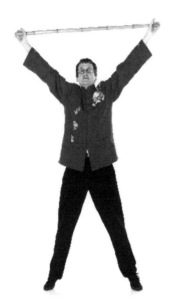

Figure 2.2

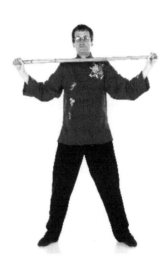

Figure 2.3

STAGE 2 METAL 金

Exhale completely as you bring the Gan down past your face, close to your body, till it reaches your chest, while simultaneously coming down from your toes and bending your knees slightly. Keep your back straight (Figure 2.4). Then inhale deeply as you push the Gan back up to the beginning stage, rising onto your toes again and stretching your body as the Gan goes as high as you can push it.

STAGE 3 WATER 水

Exhale completely as you bring the Gan down past your face, close to your body, till it reaches your navel, while coming down from your toes and bending your knees to a half-seated position (Figure 2.5). Then inhale deeply as you raise the Gan back up to the beginning stage, rising onto your toes again, stretching your body as the Gan goes as high as you can lift it.

STAGE 4 WOOD 木

Exhale completely as you lower the Gan past your face, close to your body, till it reaches your lower hip area. At the same time come down from your toes and bend the knees into a half-seated position. Then inhale deeply as you push the Gan back up to the beginning stage, rising onto your toes again, stretching your body as the Gan goes as high as you can lift it.

STAGE 5 FIRE 火

Exhale completely as you lower the Gan past your face, close to the body, till it reaches the top of your thighs. At the same time come down from your toes and bend your knees to half-seated position. Then inhale deeply as you push the Gan back up to the beginning stage, rising onto your toes again, stretching your body as the Gan goes as high as you can lift it.

FINAL STAGE YANG 阳

Exhale completely as you lower the Gan past your face, close to your body, till it reaches a few inches below the top of your thighs. At the same time come down from your toes and bend your knees into a slightly deeper half-seated position (Figure 2.6). Then inhale deeply as you raise the Gan back up to the beginning stage, rising onto your toes again and stretching your body as the Gan goes as high as you can lift it.

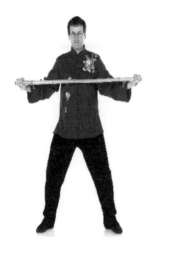 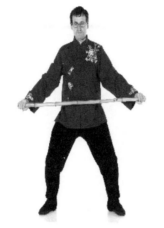 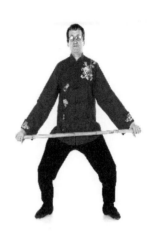

Figure 2.4   Figure 2.5   Figure 2.6

YIN 阴 TO YANG 阳

Perform the beginning stage to final stage (Figure 2.2 to Figure 2.6) missing out the intermediary stages, repeating as many times as you are able or feel comfortable doing.

Figure 2.7 shows the 'Yin to Earth' and 'Yin to Metal' stages.

ADAPTATION

As with the previous exercise, if you find it hard to stand on your toes, just move your weight to the front of your feet. You may eventually be able to raise your heels off the ground. But do not miss out this posture just because you have trouble standing on your toes or you will miss its great benefits. If you cannot lower yourself very far, just go as far as you are comfortable. You may be able to squat at a lower level after repeated practice. Although the 'ideal' is to stretch the Gan up as high as you can to the Yin position and to squat in the Yang position, individuals will have their own limit on how far they can go. With most people this 'limit' will expand with practice as the body becomes more supple and stronger. The squat in this exercise is combined with rising movements, which makes it a far more comprehensive exercise than a conventional squat.

Yin to Earth Sequence

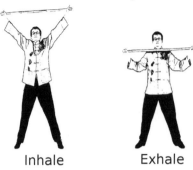

Inhale   Exhale

Yin to Metal Sequence

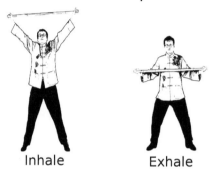

Inhale   Exhale

Figure 2.7

ENERGY ACTIVATION: STRETCHING THE PYRAMID

In all the exercises the Gan actually creates two pyramids and of course two 'tips' or vertices – one at the crown of the head (Baihui) and the other in the Perineum (Huiyin). In some exercises both these points are stimulated equally at the same time, but in most exercises there is an ebb and flow as one pyramid is passive while the other is active. In the Yin to Yang repetitions of this exercise, the Gan completely activates the dual energy centres, constantly moving Qi from the Huiyin point at the base of the spine (as the Gan is lowered from above the head) up to the Baihui point at the top of the head (when the Gan reaches the thighs). You may want to visualise fire or heat rising up your back as you perform this action. Then as you return the Gan to the beginning Yin position with the Gan above your head, you may imagine Yin cooling water flowing down the front of your body to the Huiyin point. This has a flushing and energising effect on the body as Qi is kept in steady motion. See Figure 2.8.

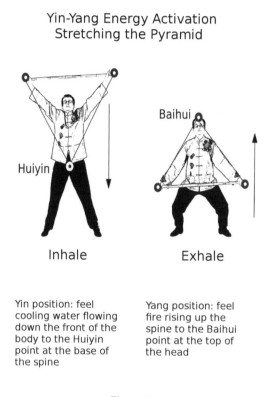

Yin-Yang Energy Activation
Stretching the Pyramid

Huiyin

Baihui

Inhale

Exhale

Yin position: feel cooling water flowing down the front of the body to the Huiyin point at the base of the spine

Yang position: feel fire rising up the spine to the Baihui point at the top of the head

Figure 2.8

Notes

As you sink, your body must be straight so that the Baihui and Huiyin points are in alignment. This is an excellent exercise for the back and one of the most beneficial for improving posture. The elbows gently lock, open and lock again as they reach the Yin and Yang positions. Hold the Gan close to your body at all times. Following on from the first exercise, you are again rising onto your toes then bending your knees. This Yin-Yang type movement enhances the coordination between body and breathing. This exercise serves as a second warm-up, easing you a little further into the swing of the routine.

From this point on you will be holding the Gan during each exercise, so instead of imagining Heavenly Qi being gathered by your open palms you can, if you wish, imagine Qi entering the ends of the Gan, flowing along it and through your hands and fingers then up your arms and then going into your body.

3 Peeling the Octopus 剥章鱼

BEGINNING STAGE YIN 阴

Stand erect with feet in a medium stance. Hold the Gan in a wide grip horizontally above your head in a line with the back of your neck (Figure 3.1). Do not rise up onto your toes at any time during this exercise. Note also that the breathing is different from the previous exercise. Each stage continues from the previous one without pause unless mentioned in the description.

STAGE 1 EARTH 土

Inhale deeply as you lower the Gan to the back of your head (Figure 3.2). Then exhale completely as you raise the Gan back up to the beginning Yin stage and stretch your arms to the fullest extent, locking your elbows. Raise the Gan as high as you can every time you return to the beginning stage.

STAGE 2 METAL 金

Inhale deeply as you lower the Gan to touch the back of your neck (Figure 3.3). Then exhale completely as you raise the Gan back up to the beginning stage and stretch your arms to the fullest extent, locking your elbows again.

STAGE 3 WATER 水

Inhale deeply as you bring the Gan down to touch the back of your shoulders (Figure 3.4). Then exhale completely as you lift the Gan back up to the beginning stage, stretching your arms to the fullest extent and locking your elbows.

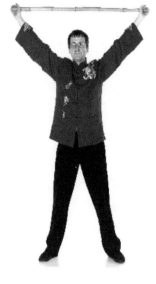

Figure 3.1

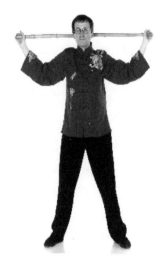

Figure 3.2

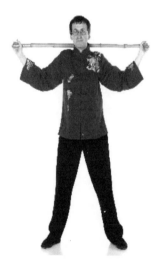

Figure 3.3

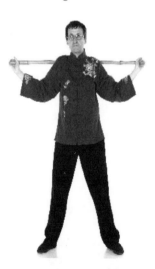

Figure 3.4

STAGE 4 WOOD 木

Inhale deeply as you lower the Gan to touch the back of your shoulder blades, releasing your grip a little (Figure 3.5). Then exhale completely as you raise the Gan back up to the beginning stage and stretch your arms to the fullest extent, locking your elbows.

STAGE 5 FIRE 火

Inhale deeply as you bring the Gan down and touch your lower back (Figure 3.6). You will have to loosen your grip slightly to adjust to the position of the Gan. Then exhale completely as you raise the Gan back up to the beginning stage, stretching your arms to the fullest extent and locking your elbows.

FINAL STAGE YANG 阳

Inhale deeply as you bring the Gan down and touch your buttocks, loosening your grip on the Gan so that you end up holding it between the thumb and forefinger. Stretch arms and lock the elbows, hesitating for an instant (Figures 3.7 and 3.8). Then exhale completely as you raise the Gan back up to the beginning stage and stretch your arms to the fullest extent and lock your elbows. Raise the Gan as high as you can every time you return to the beginning stage.

YIN 阴 TO YANG 阳

Then perform the beginning stage to the final stage (Figures 3.1 to 3.7) missing out the intermediary stages, repeating as many times as you are able or feel comfortable doing.

Figure 3.9 shows the 'Yin to Earth' and 'Yin to Water' stages.

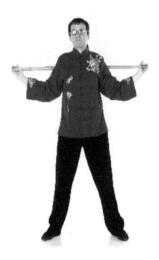

Figure 3.5

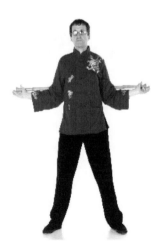

Figure 3.6

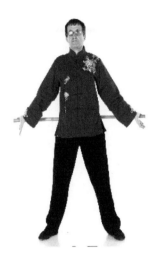

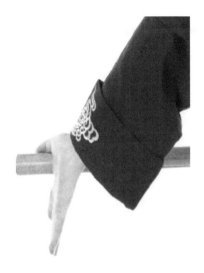

Figure 3.7   Figure 3.8

Yin to Earth Sequence

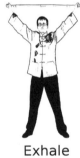

Exhale

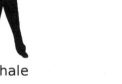

Inhale

Yin to Water Sequence

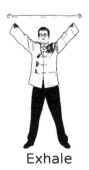

Exhale

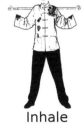

Inhale

Figure 3.9

ADAPTATION

If you are stiff in the shoulder or neck region, you may not be able to bring the Gan down much past the back of your head (or indeed lift it very high above your head). If this is the case you can use the beginner's preparation exercise, which consists of starting with the Gan on your chest then lifting it up and into the beginning Yin posture of this exercise. When you have become used to this, you can then go into the 'Inch-by-Inch' method described in Chapter 8, perhaps going only as far as the first or second stages at first, then after some weeks gradually going further down. Your practical range of movement will serve as your 'Yin' and 'Yang' stages. Repeating whatever short range of movement you are able to perform, with breathing, will bring great benefits.

ENERGY ACTIVATION: LIFTING THE PYRAMID

In the Yin to Yang repetitions, the Gan completely activates the dual energy centres, constantly moving Qi from the Huiyin point at the base of the spine (as the Gan is lowered from above and behind the head) up to the Baihui point at the top of the head (when the Gan reaches the buttocks). You may want to visualise fire or heat rising up your back as you perform this action. Then as you return the Gan above the back of your head, you may imagine Yin cooling water flowing down the front of your body to the Huiyin point. See Figure 3.10.

Notes

This exercise looks easy but from experience I have found that it is the most difficult for many people, simply because the movement of bringing the Gan down behind the head exposes many neck, shoulder and arm weaknesses. People with problems in this respect should start with the beginner's preparation as above. Muscles of the shoulders, neck, arms, chest, back and waist are exercised in particular and it is superb for improving posture and for anyone with arthritis in the upper body or who suffers from stiffness in this region.

Your hands must be precise in this exercise. When you hold the Gan between forefinger and thumb in the Yang stage, ensure that your palms are open as if to receive Heavenly Qi. Whenever you raise the Gan back up to the beginning after changing the grip, make sure you grasp it again correctly as soon as you are able to do so, making a gentle fist. At the Yin-Yang repetition stage, be aware that the opening and closing of your hands is synchronised with your breathing. This exercise is excellent not only for people with shoulder, neck and upper body problems but also for 'tasking' the hands, wrists and fingers as well as gently working the back, shoulders and neck. Keep the Gan close to the back of your body and keep it horizontal at all times. Do not let one side drop lower than the other. Your lower body must be fixed and your legs straight and held firmly in place. There is no need to lock knees but do not bend them too much. I have found that a gentle locking of the knees gives the stability required for this exercise.

Yin-Yang Energy Activation
Lifting the Pyramid

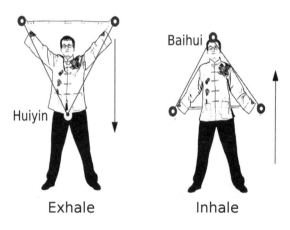

Exhale · Inhale

Yin position: feel cooling water flowing down the front of the body to the Huiyin point at the base of the spine

Yang position: feel fire rising up the spine to the Baihui point at the top of the head

Figure 3.10

81

4 Twisting the Snake 扭蛇

BEGINNING STAGE YIN 阴

Stand erect, feet in a medium width stance, holding the Gan in a wide grip straight out in front of you, elbows locked, in line with your shoulders (Figure 4.1). Each stage continues from the previous one without pause unless mentioned in the description.

STAGE 1 EARTH 土 (RIGHT SIDE)

Inhale deeply as you swing your right arm up and around towards your left side, raising it so that your right hand goes up and over the top of your head (Figure 4.2). Continue moving the Gan around behind you, touching your neck briefly (same as Figure 3.3). Then exhale completely as you keep the Gan moving and roll it around your neck, continuing to bring it back to the front of the body by raising your left arm up overhead to the right side (Figure 4.3). In a continuous movement bring the Gan back to the beginning stage (Figure 4.1).

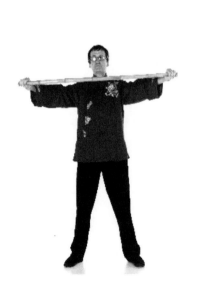
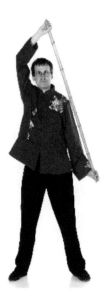
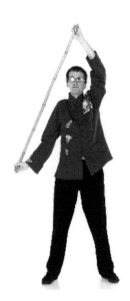

Figure 4.1   Figure 4.2   Figure 4.3

STAGE 1 EARTH 土 (LEFT SIDE)

Repeat the stage in the opposite direction with your left arm taking the lead (start by swinging your left arm up around the right side).

STAGE 2 METAL 金 (RIGHT SIDE)

Inhale deeply as you circle the Gan again from the beginning stage over your left side, this time rolling it around your shoulders (same as Figure 3.4). Then exhale completely as you continue bringing the Gan back over the right side of your head and right shoulder until you are holding it straight out in front of you again in the beginning stage.

STAGE 2 METAL 金 (LEFT SIDE)

Repeat this stage in the opposite direction (swinging your left arm up around the right side).

STAGE 3 WATER 水 (RIGHT SIDE)

Inhale deeply as you circle the Gan from the beginning stage over your left shoulder and bring it down to make brief contact with the upper shoulder blades (slightly higher than Figure 3.5). Then exhale completely as you continue bringing the Gan over the right side of your head and right shoulder until you are again holding it in front of you in the beginning stage.

STAGE 3 WATER 水 (LEFT SIDE)

Repeat this stage in the opposite direction (swinging your left arm up around the right side).

STAGE 4 WOOD 木 (RIGHT SIDE)

Inhale deeply as you circle the Gan from the beginning stage over your left shoulder and bring it down close to the body to briefly touch your middle back (slightly higher than Figure 3.6). From this stage to the final stage, you will have to change your grip slightly so that by the final Yang stage, the

Gan is held between thumb and forefinger. Then exhale completely as you continue bringing the Gan back over the right side of your head and right shoulder until you are again holding it in front of you in the beginning stage.

STAGE 4 WOOD 木 (LEFT SIDE)

Repeat this stage in the opposite direction (swinging your left arm up around the right side).

STAGE 5 FIRE 火 (RIGHT SIDE)

Inhale deeply as you circle the Gan from the beginning stage over your left shoulder and bring it down close to the body to lightly touch the lower back (same as Figure 3.6). Then exhale completely as you continue bringing the Gan back over the right side of your head and right shoulder until you are again holding it in front of you in the beginning stage.

STAGE 5 FIRE 火 (LEFT SIDE)

Repeat this stage in the opposite direction (swinging your left arm up around the right side).

FINAL STAGE YANG 阳 (RIGHT SIDE)

Inhale deeply as you circle the Gan from the beginning stage over your left shoulder and bring it down close to the body to the final stage resting against the buttocks – which is identical to the final stage of the 'Peeling the Octopus' exercise (same as Figure 3.7). Stretch arms and lock the elbows, hesitating for an instant. Then exhale completely as you continue bringing the Gan back over the right side of your head and right shoulder until you are again holding it in front of you in the beginning stage.

FINAL STAGE YANG 阳 (LEFT SIDE)

Repeat this stage in the opposite direction (swinging your left arm up around the right side).

BEGINNING STAGE YIN 阴 TO FINAL STAGE YANG 阳

Perform the beginning stage to the final stage, repeating as many times as you are able or feel comfortable doing.

Figure 4.4 shows the Yin to Earth stage, right side.

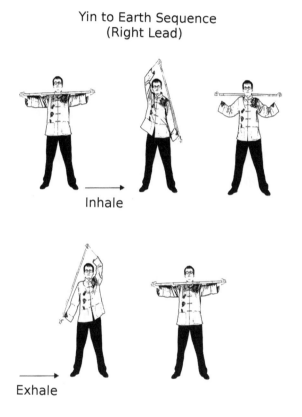

Yin to Earth Sequence
(Right Lead)

Inhale

Exhale

Figure 4.4

ADAPTATION

As with the 'Peeling the Octopus' exercise, people with stiff shoulders may only be able to bring the Gan around the back of their heads. If so, this becomes the 'Yang' stage and there is still great benefit to be obtained from even performing this sequence. Perseverance will certainly bring increased mobility and suppleness in this important region of the body.

ENERGY ACTIVATION: CIRCLING THE PYRAMID

This exercise activates the Huiyin point at the base of the spine from left and right lateral angles and allows Qi to flow up to reach the Baihui point at the top of your head (when the Gan reaches your buttocks). You may want to visualise fire or heat rising up your back as you perform this action. Then as you return the Gan to the front of your body you may imagine Yin cooling water flowing down the front of your body to the Huiyin point. See Figure 4.5.

**Yin-Yang Energy Activation
Circling the Pyramid (Right Side)**

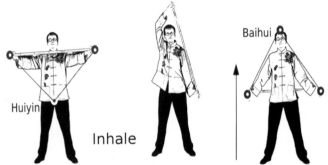

From the beginning position, feel fire rising up the spine to the Baihui point at the top of the head at the Yang position

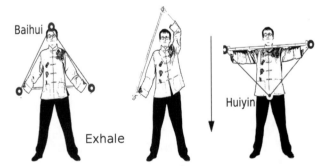

From the Yang position, feel cooling water flowing down the front of the body to the Huiyin point at the base of the spine as you return to the beginning

Figure 4.5

Notes

This exercise is everyone's instant favourite. All the health professionals I have shown it to have commented that it is the perfect range of movements for a wide range of shoulder, upper back, lower back, arm, wrist and neck complaints. It is also the exercise that elicits the most positive response from beginners because of the easy windmill-like movement of the arms. Like the previous exercise this is excellent not only for shoulder, arm, neck and upper body problems but also for the back, including lower back problems and even hip conditions. But although this exercise looks easy, some coordination is required in the hands in the later stages, opening and closing them at the correct points; ensure that your hands clasp the Gan in a light 'fist' each time you return the Gan to the Yin stage, and open them when the Gan is lowered around the lower rear of your body. As in 'Peeling the Octopus', this opening and closing in the final Yang repetitions – coordinating with the breathing – creates a relaxing cyclic effect. As with the previous exercise there is no need to lock knees but do not bend them too much. I have found that a gentle locking of the knees gives the stability required for this exercise.

5 Twitching the Dragon's Tail 龙尾抽搐

BEGINNING STAGE YIN 阴

Stand erect, feet in a medium-width stance, holding the Gan in a wide grip while resting it against the back of your shoulders (Figure 5.1). Your back should be kept straight, your knees locked and chin up. This exercise is for the upper body and your lower body must not assist. Look directly in front of you. Do not bend forwards during this exercise. Each stage continues from the previous one without pause unless mentioned in the description.

STAGE 1 EARTH 土 (WORKING THE LEFT SIDE)

Inhale deeply.

Twist – Exhale completely as you move the Gan to the right by twisting your left arm and upper body a few inches to the right. Make sure your head keeps facing directly forwards (Figure 5.2). Then inhale deeply as you return to the beginning Yin stage, holding the position for a second.

Bend – Exhale completely as you bend your upper body to the left a few inches, as if you intend to point the left end of the Gan towards the floor (Figure 5.3). Inhale deeply as you return to the beginning stage, holding the position for a second.

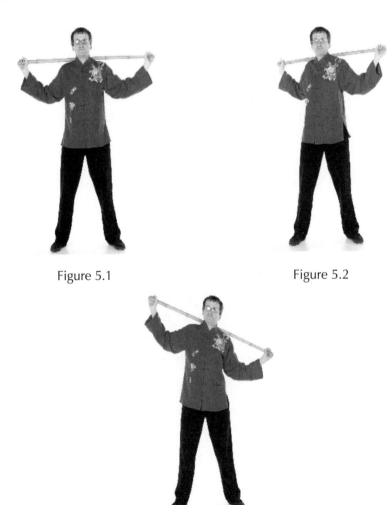

Figure 5.1   Figure 5.2

Figure 5.3

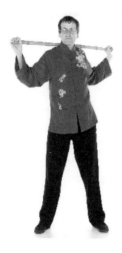
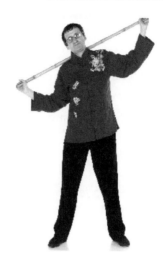

| Figure 5.4 | Figure 5.5 |

STAGE 1 EARTH 土 (WORKING THE RIGHT SIDE)

Twist – Exhale completely as you move the Gan to the left by twisting your right arm and upper body a few inches to the left. Make sure you keep your head facing directly forwards (Figure 5.4). Then inhale deeply as you return to the beginning stage, holding the position for a second.

Bend – Exhale completely as you bend your upper body to the right a few inches, as if you intend to point the right end of the Gan towards the floor (Figure 5.5). Inhale deeply as you return to the beginning stage, holding the position for a second.

STAGE 2 METAL 金 (WORKING THE LEFT SIDE)

Twist – Exhale completely as you twist your left arm and shoulders a little further to the right than Stage 1, keeping your head facing forwards. Then inhale deeply as you return to the beginning stage, holding the position for a second.

Bend – Exhale completely as you bend your upper body to your left side as you did in Stage 1, only a little further. Then inhale deeply as you return to the beginning stage, holding the position for a second.

STAGE 2 METAL 金 (WORKING THE RIGHT SIDE)

Twist – Exhale completely as you twist your right arm and shoulders to the left as you did in Stage 1, only a little further. Keep your head facing forwards. Then inhale deeply as you return to the beginning stage, holding the position for a second.

Bend – Exhale completely as you bend your upper body to your right side as you did in Stage 1, only a little further. Then inhale deeply as you return to the beginning stage, holding the position for a second.

STAGE 2 WATER 水 TO FINAL STAGE YANG 阳 (WORKING THE LEFT AND RIGHT SIDES)

Continue twisting and bending in this way, a little further each time till you reach the left side Yang twist (Figure 5.6) and left side Yang bend (Figure 5.7), and right side Yang twist (Figure 5.8) and right side Yang bend (Figure 5.9).

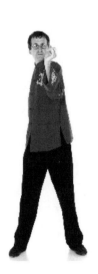

Figure 5.6

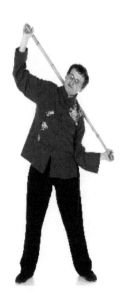

Figure 5.7

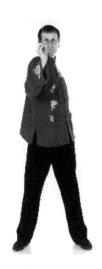
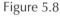
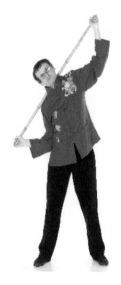

Figure 5.8   Figure 5.9

BEGINNING STAGE YIN 阴 TO FINAL STAGE YANG 阳

Perform the Yin stage to Yang stage, missing out the intermediary stages and repeating as many times as you are able or feel comfortable doing.

Figure 5.10 shows the Yin to Earth stage (left side).

ADAPTATION

Many people will not be able to reach the featured final positions. If you cannot reach them, go as far as you are able.

Yin to Earth Sequence (Left)

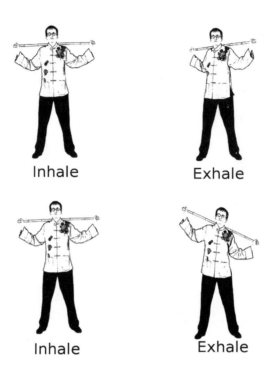

Figure 5.10

ENERGY ACTIVATION: TWISTING THE PYRAMID

In both the twist and the bend, the Gan primarily activates the Huiyin point at the base of the spine, which allows Qi to flow up and throughout the body. You may want to visualise fire or heat rising up your back as you perform the bends and twists, then as you return to the beginning Yin position, you may imagine Yin or cooling water flowing down the front of the body to the Huiyin point. See Figure 5.11.

Yin-Yang Energy Activation
Twisting the Pyramid

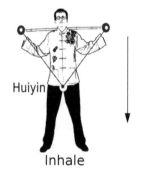

Huiyin

Inhale

At the beginning, Yin position, feel cooling water flowing down the front of the body to the Huiyin point at the base of the spine

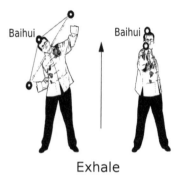

Baihui   Baihui

Exhale

Going into the Yang positions of the BEND and TWIST (right side shown here), feel fire rising up the spine to the Baihui point at the top of the head

Figure 5.11

Notes

This is the most misunderstood exercise in the whole routine. On superficial overview it might look as if we are performing one of those broom-across-the-shoulders body swinging exercises. But we are *not* turning the whole body and head. This exercise is far more subtle and potent. Its aim is not only to stretch muscles of the torso but also to massage internal organs and to do this, the waist and hips region must not move. The most important aspect in the twist is keeping the head and lower body (everything below the waist) absolutely still and facing the front (aligning the Baihui and Huiyin points, which should be still). The only parts of the body that move are the shoulders, arms and upper torso. This exercise looks 'external' and physical but it is one of the most internal and subtle in the whole routine because it requires control and focus to perform correctly. In order to move only your

93

arms and shoulders, you must employ focus and it takes a long time to learn because the instinct is for the waist and the head to move with the shoulders. You will discover that this is essentially an 'internal' type of movement. In the first few stages of this exercise, it is absolutely essential that you do not attempt to twist or bend too far too soon. Even fit people may take months to reach the Yang stages shown in this book. Just go as far as you are able and you will experience the great benefit of this exercise. This exercise also strengthens the arms because the aim is to rest the Gan *lightly* on the back of the shoulders and so the arms must take some of the weight. Be careful not to 'rest' your arms and pull the Gan down into your shoulders creating a downward pressure which is not good for the shoulders or back. And never *ever* perform this exercise resting your wrists on the top of the Gan (like some 'broomstick-across-the-shoulders' exercises you may have seen). This would cut off circulation of both blood and Qi in your hands and be injurious to your back and shoulders. This exercise particularly targets not only the muscles of the side trunk – the obliques – but also hips, buttocks, legs, arms, neck, shoulders and back. The twists are superb for the upper back and shoulder blades. It is advantageous to keep the knees locked in this exercise. This gives the legs a good stretch and provides stability.

6 Bowing 鞠躬

FRONT BEGINNING STAGE YIN 阴

Stand erect with feet in a medium-wide stance. Hold the Gan with a wide grip, resting it gently on the upper chest. Keep the knees locked and legs straight at all times (Figure 6.1). Each stage continues from the previous one without pause unless mentioned in the description.

FRONT STAGE 1 EARTH 土

Exhale completely as you bring the Gan down and bend your upper body slightly, the Gan finishing by touching the top of the thighs (Figure 6.2). Then inhale deeply as you return to the front beginning stage.

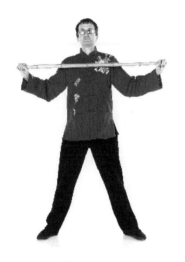

Figure 6.1

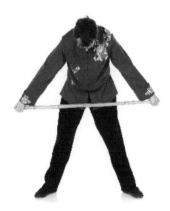

Figure 6.2

LEFT BEGINNING STAGE YIN 阴

Turn your upper body so that it is completely facing the left. Hold for one second (Figure 6.3).

LEFT STAGE 1 EARTH 土

Then exhale completely as you bring the Gan down, bending your upper body slightly, the Gan finishing by touching the side of your upper left thigh (Figure 6.4). Then inhale deeply as you return to the left beginning stage. Hold this position for a second then twist back to the front beginning stage.

FRONT STAGE 2 METAL 金

Exhale completely as you bring the Gan down and bend over from your waist, the Gan finishing by touching the middle of your thighs (Figure 6.5). Then inhale deeply as you return to the front beginning stage.

RIGHT BEGINNING STAGE YIN 阴

Turn your upper body so that it is completely facing the right. Hold for one second (Figure 6.6).

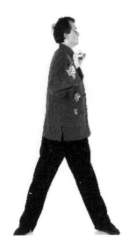

Figure 6.3

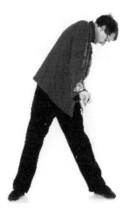

Figure 6.4

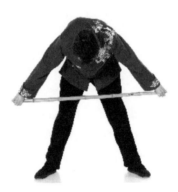

Figure 6.5

RIGHT STAGE 1 EARTH 土

Exhale completely as you bring the Gan down and bend your upper body slightly, the Gan finishing by touching the side of your upper right thigh (Figure 6.7). Then inhale deeply as you return to the right beginning stage. Hold this position for a second then twist back to the front beginning stage.

FRONT STAGE 3 WATER 水

Exhale completely as you bring the Gan down, bending from your waist, the Gan finishing about level with your knees (Figure 6.8). Then inhale deeply as you return to the beginning stage.

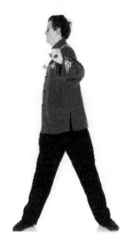

Figure 6.6

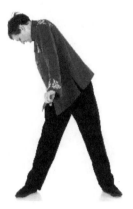

Figure 6.7

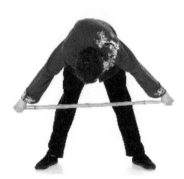

Figure 6.8

FRONT, LEFT AND RIGHT STAGE 3 WOOD 木 TO FINAL STAGE YANG 阳

Continue using the same method – first left side, then front and right – to bring the Gan a little further down your legs each time, exhaling when bending and inhaling when returning to the beginning stages. In the final stages, aim to touch the Gan against your ankles at the front (Figure 6.9) and the lower leg on the right and left sides (Figures 6.10 and 6.11).

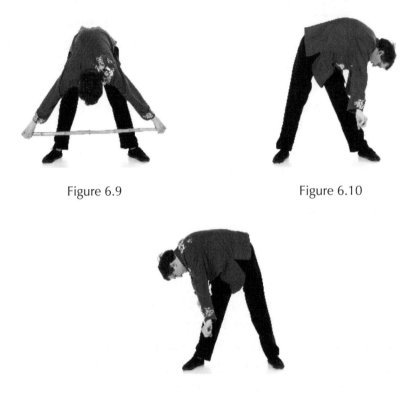

Figure 6.9   Figure 6.10

Figure 6.11

BEGINNING STAGE YIN 阴 TO FINAL STAGE YANG 阳

Perform the beginning stage to the final stage – front, left and right – missing out the intermediary stages and repeating as many times as you are able or feel comfortable doing.

Figure 6.12 shows the Yin to Earth stage.

Yin to Earth Sequence (Left)

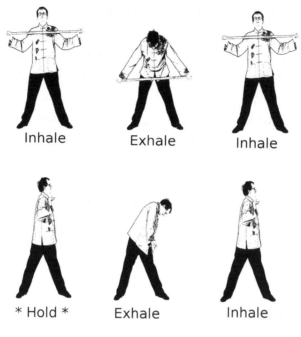

Figure 6.12

ADAPTATION

For anyone with back problems and unable to reach the lower positions in any direction, I advise simply bending a few inches for the entire stages. After you have built up confidence and if you have not experienced any problems, you can gradually, with each session, bend a little further forwards.

ENERGY ACTIVATION: BOWING THE PYRAMID

The bending, twisting and stretching movements activate the dual energy centres and moves Qi from the Huiyin point at the base of the spine to the Baihui point at the top of the head. This refreshes and energises the whole body. You may want to visualise fire or heat rising up your back as you perform the bends, then as you return the Gan to the beginning Yin position (with the Gan across your chest), you may imagine Yin cooling water flowing down the front of your body to the Huiyin point. See Figure 6.13.

Yin-Yang Energy Activation
Bowing the Pyramid

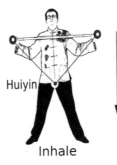

At the beginning Yin position, feel cooling water flowing down the front of the body to the Huiyin point at the base of the spine

Huiyin

Inhale

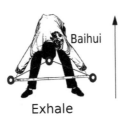

Going into the Yang position, feel fire rising up the spine to the Baihui point at the top of the head

Baihui

Exhale

Figure 6.13

Notes

Although this exercise primarily exercises the lower body – particularly the legs, hips, buttocks and waist – the entire back, shoulders, arms and neck also receive very beneficial exercise. Make sure you straighten your arms (lock your elbows) before you bend fully and keep the Gan against your body because the Gan is your measure and ruler, ensuring that you do not bend too far too quickly. *Do not* use your arms to push down with the Gan and *do not* hold the Gan out away from your body. Your waist should lead in bending, not your arms. This exercise more than any other shows how the Gan assists and supports the body performing an exercise that would be difficult to do 'empty handed'. Think of your body as a building and the Gan as the scaffolding. It is important that your shoulders are in alignment with the Gan. Holding it against your upper chest maintains the support. Do not let the Gan 'float' away from your body.

7 Greeting the Traveller 欢迎旅客

BEGINNING STAGE YIN 阴

Stand erect, feet close together, holding the Gan in a wide grip lightly over the back of the shoulders. Arch your back *slightly* backwards, keeping your legs straight (knees locked) at all times. Your chin must be kept up and your head tilted back, eyes looking up, throughout this exercise. You start by looking at the ceiling or sky directly above you (Figure 7.1).

STAGE 1 EARTH 土

Exhale completely as you slowly bend forwards from your hips a few inches, keeping your back arched and head high (Figure 7.2). Then inhale deeply as you return to the beginning stage.

STAGE 2 METAL 金

Exhale completely as you slowly bend forwards from your hips a few inches further than Stage 1, keeping your back arched and head high (Figure 7.3). Then inhale deeply as you return to the beginning stage.

STAGE 3 WATER 水 TO FINAL STAGE YANG 阳

Exhale completely as you slowly bend forwards from your hips a little further each time, keeping your back slightly arched and head high; the final stage will vary according to each person. Fit people should be able to reach to within about ten degrees above the level of their waist or even a little further (see Figure 7.4). Then inhale deeply as you return to the beginning stage.

BEGINNING STAGE YIN 阴 TO FINAL STAGE YANG 阳

Perform the beginning stage to the final stage slowly, missing out the intermediary stages and repeating as many times as you are able or feel comfortable doing. Remember to keep your head up, eyes looking up and back slightly arched at all times. Never look down at the floor during this exercise. Hold your last Yang stage position for a count of three while holding your breath, then slowly rise, inhaling, to the beginning Yin stage, then count to three. Then exhale slowly.

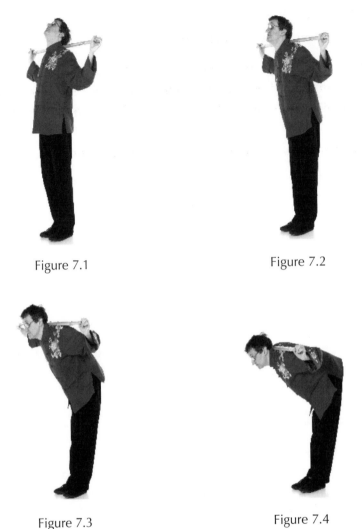

Figure 7.1

Figure 7.2

Figure 7.3

Figure 7.4

ADAPTATION

This can seem like an alarming exercise but if you follow the directions carefully, it will do wonders for a range of back problems. If you are unable – or feel that you are unable – to reach the lower positions, I advise simply bending a few inches for the entire stages. After you have built up confidence and have not experienced any problems, you can gradually, with each session, bend a little further forwards.

ENERGY ACTIVATION: GREETING THE PYRAMID

In the elemental stages Qi is focused on the back, waist and legs, but in the Yin to Yang sequence Qi moves upwards and gives a flushing sensation throughout the body as it moves from the Huiyin point at the base of the spine to the Baihui point at the top of the head. You may want to visualise fire or heat rising up your back as you perform the bends, then, as you return to the beginning Yin position, you may imagine Yin cooling water flowing down the front of your body to the Huiyin point. See Figure 7.5.

Yin-Yang Energy Activation
Greeting the Pyramid

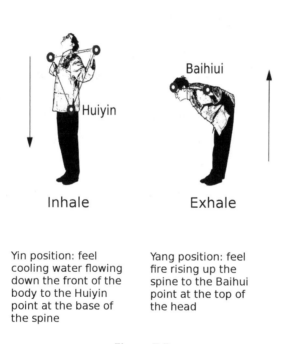

Inhale   Exhale

Yin position: feel cooling water flowing down the front of the body to the Huiyin point at the base of the spine

Yang position: feel fire rising up the spine to the Baihui point at the top of the head

Figure 7.5

Notes

This exercise is excellent for the entire back region, waist, hips, buttocks, legs, chest, neck, chin and the facial muscles. The graduated stages method combined with the slow pace protects and strengthens muscles in your back as you go through this exercise. People with a range of back problems should feel quite comfortable performing it as long as they follow instructions correctly. As with 'Twitching the Dragon's Tail', do not press down on your shoulders with the Gan at any time; keep it light. In the first few stages of this exercise you may feel energy concentrating on your back, legs and waist. In the final Yin-Yang sequence you may feel the energy flow to the top of your head and all around your body.

8 Search for the Hatchet 找柴刀

BEGINNING STAGE YIN 阴

Stand erect, feet between medium and wide stance, your back slightly arched backwards. For this posture you need to hold the Gan behind your back against the backs of your thighs. This exercise uses a different grip. Place your hands about a foot from the ends of the Gan with knuckles facing forwards. The elbows and knees are kept locked at all times (Figure 8.1).

STAGE 1 EARTH 土

Exhale completely as you bend forwards slightly, lifting the Gan away from your body (Figure 8.2). Then inhale deeply as you return to the beginning stage, keeping your back slightly arched, with your head high and eyes looking up.

STAGE 2 METAL 金

Exhale completely as you bend forwards a little further than Stage 1, lifting the Gan a bit further away from your body (Figure 8.3). Then inhale deeply as you return to the beginning stage.

STAGE 3 WATER 水

Exhale completely as you bend forwards further as in Figure 8.4, eyes looking ahead, chin up, and push the Gan up behind you a bit further. Then inhale deeply as you return to the beginning stage.

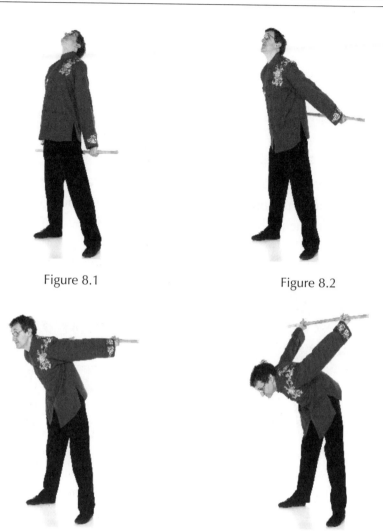

Figure 8.1

Figure 8.2

Figure 8.3

Figure 8.4

STAGE 4 WOOD 木

Exhale completely as you bend forwards a little further than Stage 3, eyes looking ahead, chin up as high as you can, and push the Gan up behind you above your head (Figure 8.5). Then inhale deeply as you return to the beginning stage.

STAGE 5 FIRE 火

Exhale completely as you bend forwards a little further than Stage 4 and push the Gan above your head. Then inhale deeply as you return to the beginning stage.

FINAL STAGE YANG 阳

Exhale completely as you bend forwards as far as you can and stretch the Gan right up over your head and out towards the front, eyes now looking at the floor (Figure 8.6). Then inhale deeply as you return to the beginning stage.

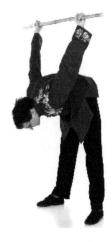

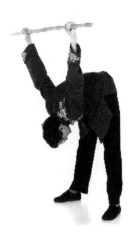

Figure 8.5   Figure 8.6

BEGINNING STAGE YIN 阴 TO FINAL STAGE YANG 阳

Repeat, slowly, missing out the various stages, as many times as you are able. Hold the last final stage position for a slow count of four after exhaling then slowly rise up back to the beginning stage, inhaling deeply. Then exhale completely and slowly.

ADAPTATION

This is another exercise that looks rather alarming but if you follow the directions carefully, it will do wonders for a range of back, leg and arm circulation problems. If you are unable to reach the lower positions, I advise bending forwards to Stage 2 or 3 (doing so in five slow stages accompanied with deep breathing as described). After you have built up confidence and if you have not experienced any problems, you can gradually, with each session, bend a little further.

ENERGY ACTIVATION: THRUSTING THE PYRAMID

In this exercise Qi constantly moves back and forth from the Huiyin point at the base of the spine to the Baihui point at the top of the head, which stimulates the entire body, mind and spirit, making it a fantastic energy activator. You may want to visualise fire or heat rising up your back as you perform the bends, then as you return the Gan to the beginning Yin position, you may imagine Yin cooling water flowing down the front of the body to the Huiyin point. See Figure 8.7.

Yin-Yang Energy Activation
Thrusting the Pyramid

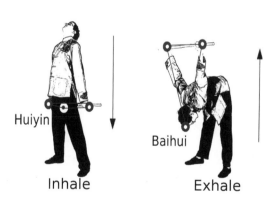

Huiyin

Baihui

Inhale

Exhale

Yin position: feel cooling water flowing down the front of the body to the Huiyin point at the base of the spine

Yang position: feel fire rising up the spine to the Baihui point at the top of the head

Figure 8.7

Notes

This exercise works the entire back region, arms, waist, hips, buttocks, shoulders, neck, legs and chest. Like the previous exercise, this is excellent for firming the chin and facial muscles. Flabby, soft muscles in the neck, face and the back of the arms will be toned and firmed with this exercise. You are creating a narrower pyramid with this exercise with more intense focus on the vertex (Baihui and Huiyin points).

9 Horse Stance on a Tightrope 绳索马式

BEGINNING STAGE YIN 阴

Stand erect, feet in a very wide stance with toes pointing *outwards* to the sides of the body so that your heels face each other. The angle of the toes should be 180 degrees, as if you are on a tightrope. Hold the Gan lightly against your shoulders at the back in a wide grip. Keep your back straight and look directly forwards throughout this exercise (Figure 9.1).

STAGE 1 EARTH 土

Exhale completely, arch your back slightly backwards as you slowly bend your knees a few inches. Then inhale deeply as you slowly return to the beginning Yin stage, locking your knees (Figure 9.2).

STAGE 2 METAL 金 TO FINAL STAGE YANG 阳

Continue to go down a little further with each stage, locking your knees each time you return to the beginning position, till you reach the Yang stage when you will be in an almost fully seated position – or as if you are about to sit in a chair (Figure 9.3).

BEGINNING STAGE YIN 阴 TO FINAL STAGE YANG 阳

After the various stages you can go from the beginning stage to the final stage, missing out the intermediary stages and repeating as many times as you are able – *slowly*. On the last repetition hold the Yang position for a slow count of four while you hold your breath. Then slowly rise up to the beginning stage, inhaling slowly.

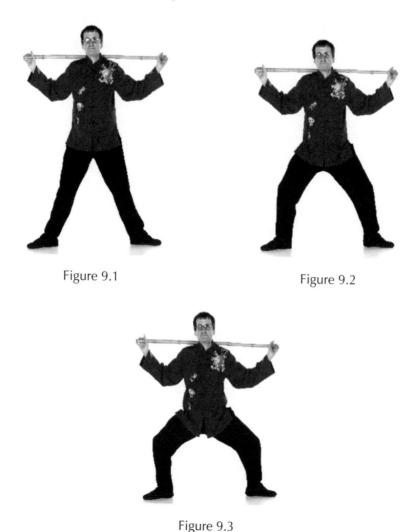

Figure 9.1   Figure 9.2

Figure 9.3

ADAPTATION

The 'Inch-by-Inch' method described in Chapter 8 is essential for everyone in this exercise. Most people will not be able to place their feet in the correct position and so can perform the exercise with the toes facing as far out as they can, gradually increasing the angle over weeks and months of practice.

ENERGY ACTIVATION: HACKING THE PYRAMID

The exercise activates stored Qi from the Huiyin point at the base of the spine and moves it throughout the lower part of the body and legs. In the Yin to Yang sequence the Qi moves to the upper body and the Baihui point at the top of the head. You may want to visualise fire or heat rising up your back as you sink, then as you return to the beginning Yin position you may imagine Yin cooling water flowing down the front of the body to the Huiyin point. See Figure 9.4.

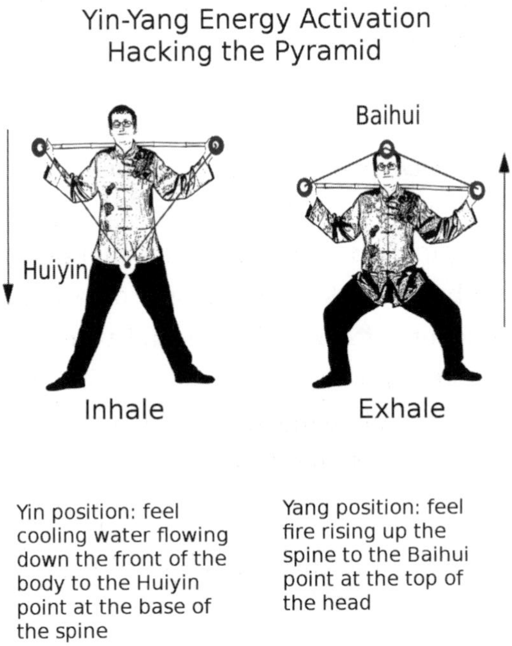

Yin-Yang Energy Activation
Hacking the Pyramid

Baihui

Huiyin

Inhale

Exhale

Yin position: feel cooling water flowing down the front of the body to the Huiyin point at the base of the spine

Yang position: feel fire rising up the spine to the Baihui point at the top of the head

Figure 9.4

Notes

This exercise targets the entire back, hips, waist, buttocks and all of the legs, particularly the inner thighs. The legs receive a complete workout and this makes this exercise the ideal gentle cardiovascular workout. Never sink too far in the final Yang position and remember that your breathing is leading the movement. This is one of the best exercises there is for developing balance and correct posture. With the feet in their outward position, it is impossible to descend leaning forwards or backwards; your body is forced to sink in a straight line. The gradual nature, slowness and repetition of the squat ensures that muscles in the back are gently stretched and that the body is aligned perfectly (in particular the Baihui and Huiyin points). This exercise is also a fantastic therapy for people who have weak knees and a wide range of knee conditions. It strengthens the whole knee area and the entire leg muscles – particularly the hamstrings – and loosens the hips. Because of the position of the feet, there is much less stress on the knees than conventional squats.

10 The Tiger Springs 老虎跳

Right Leg Lead

Go through every stage with your right leg taking the lead.

BEGINNING STAGE YIN 阴

Stand erect, feet in a medium stance. Hold the Gan high against your chest in a wide grip. Keep your back straight and look directly forwards throughout this exercise. Keep your elbows high, slightly above the Gan if possible (Figure 10.1).

STAGE 1 EARTH 土

Exhale completely as you thrust out the Gan high as you step forwards with your right leg, bending the right knee, slightly bending the rear left knee, and leaning your body away from the Gan. Then inhale deeply as you quickly step back with the right foot, returning to the beginning stage, straightening both legs.

STAGE 2 METAL 金

Exhale completely as you thrust out the Gan high as you step forwards with your right leg, bending the right knee a little more and bending the rear left knee a little more as you lean your body away from the Gan. Then inhale deeply as you quickly step back with the right foot, returning to the beginning stage, straightening both legs.

STAGE 3 WATER 水 TO FINAL STAGE YANG 阳

Continue to bend your legs a little further each time you step forwards with the right foot, till you reach the final Yang stage where your right knee should be completely bent and your rear left knee touching the floor (Figure 10.2).

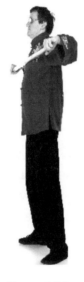
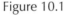
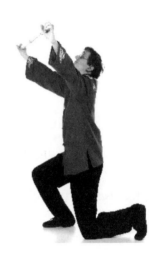

Figure 10.1   Figure 10.2

BEGINNING STAGE YIN 阴 TO FINAL STAGE YANG 阳

Miss out the intermediate stages and repeat the beginning stage to the final stage as many times as you are able.

Left Leg Lead

Now repeat the whole exercise on the left side, going through all the stages, but this time your *left* leg takes the lead.

ENERGY ACTIVATION: LUNGING THE PYRAMID

This exercise activates the dual energy centres, constantly moving Qi from the Huiyin point at the base of the spine to the Baihui point at the top of the head. Your body is kept constantly stimulated by the steady motion. You may want to visualise fire or heat rising up your back as you step forwards to perform the lunge, then as you return to the beginning Yin position you may imagine Yin cooling water flowing down the front of the body to the Huiyin point. See Figure 10.3.

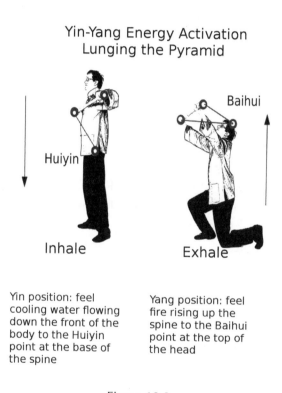

Yin-Yang Energy Activation
Lunging the Pyramid

Baihui

Huiyin

Inhale

Exhale

Yin position: feel cooling water flowing down the front of the body to the Huiyin point at the base of the spine

Yang position: feel fire rising up the spine to the Baihui point at the top of the head

Figure 10.3

ADAPTATION

It may take some people weeks or months to get to the final Yang stage (with rear knee on the floor); others will never be able to get to this position. But the important thing is to go as far as your body will allow, while keeping the posture as much as possible.

Notes

Like the previous exercise, this primarily exercises the legs – but when you learn to do this correctly you will feel significant benefit in your arms, shoulders, neck, chest, waist, hips and back. This is the only exercise in the entire routine that can be said to involve coordination to a significant degree. It is a superbly safe and effective exercise because the weight is distributed between both legs 50:50. It is a great stretch for the hamstrings and opens the hip joints and builds stamina. It is also the most effective cardiovascular exercise in the routine. The lunging motion increases circulation in the legs and lower body, while the arms, shoulders and back are worked and stretched. Your movements should be smooth and coordinated, not jerky and fast. Again breathing controls the speed.

Floor Exercises

If performing the exercises indoors on a carpet there is no need for an exercise mat. If you are practising in an area with a hard surface I recommend using an exercise mat. Local sports shops or department stores stock them, but it may be more economical to use an old mat or rug of your own.

11 Row the Boat 划船

BEGINNING STAGE YIN 阴

Sit on the floor, knees bent and slightly apart, heels together. Hold the Gan high against your chest in a wide grip, elbows up. Keep your chin tucked into your neck, and your back and shoulders rounded at all times in this exercise. Lean back to approximately a 45 degree angle; never lean further back than this (Figure 11.1).

STAGE 1 EARTH 土

Exhale completely as you bring your upper body forwards and push the Gan forwards to touch your knees (Figure 11.2). Then inhale deeply as you bring the Gan back to the beginning stage as if you are rowing a boat, careful to keep your chin in.

STAGE 2 METAL 金

Exhale completely as you bring your upper body forwards and push the Gan forwards a few inches below your knees. Then inhale deeply as you bring the Gan back to the beginning Yin stage again, careful to keep your chin in.

STAGE 3 WATER 水 TO FINAL STAGE YANG 阳

Continue to stretch the Gan a little further each time until you get to your ankles at the final stage (Figure 11.3).

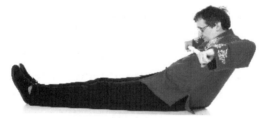

Figure 11.1

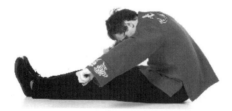

Figure 11.2

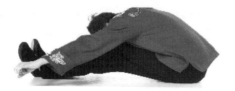

Figure 11.3

BEGINNING STAGE YIN 阴 TO FINAL STAGE YANG 阳

Miss out the various stages and repeat the beginning stage to the final stage as many times as you are able. At the end of your last repetition, when returning to the Yin stage, hold your position for a count of six.

ADAPTATION

If you find it difficult to lean into a 45 degree angle, sit straight and then go back a few inches as far as you are comfortable. And of course you bend forwards only as far as is comfortable for you.

ENERGY ACTIVATION: SETTING THE PYRAMID

The rowing and stretching movements of this exercise activate the dual energy centres, constantly moving Qi from the Huiyin point at the base of the spine to the Baihui point at the top of the head. You may want to visualise fire or heat rising up your back as you perform the bend, then as you return to the beginning Yin position with the Gan on your upper chest, you may imagine Yin cooling water flowing down the front of your body to the Huiyin point. See Figure 11.4.

Notes

This exercise targets the shoulders, neck, chest, entire back, waist, hips, buttocks and legs. It will trim the waistline by toning and firming muscles in your midsection and stretch muscles in the legs and hips, and if you can reach the final Yang position as demonstrated in his book, it will tone and firm your arms, shoulders, hips and legs. It is also an excellent gentle massage for people with back problems. Set a slow and comfortable pace. The fact that this is a 'floor exercise' does not mean that it should be treated any differently from the standing exercises. Be relaxed and move with your breathing. Do not deliberately tense the muscles and relax as much as you can. 'Row the Boat' is much safer and vastly superior to its modern Western equivalents, the 'sit-up' and 'crunch'.

Yin-Yang Energy Activation
Setting the Pyramid

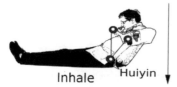

Yin position: feel cooling water flowing down the front of the body to the Huiyin point at the base of the spine

Inhale   Huiyin

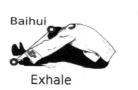

Yang position: feel fire rising up the spine to the Baihui point at the top of the head

Baihui

Exhale

Figure 11.4

12 The Rocking Bear 晃动熊

BEGINNING STAGE YIN 阴

Sit on the floor, knees bent and legs as wide apart as you can place them. Hold the Gan high against your chest in a wide grip, elbows up. Keep your chin tucked into your neck and your back and shoulders rounded at all times in this exercise. Lean back to approximately a 45 degree angle; never lean further back than this. This exercise has the same beginning posture as 'Row the Boat' except that the legs are wide. Remember to keep your elbows high (Figure 12.1).

STAGE 1 EARTH 土

Exhale completely as you bring your body forwards and twist to the right so that your left hand touches your right knee (Figure 12.2). Then inhale deeply as you bring the Gan back to the beginning stage. Then exhale completely as you bring your body forwards and twist to the left so that your right hand touches your left knee. Then inhale deeply as you bring the Gan back to the beginning stage. Each stage consists of a left and right forward bend with your hands touching the opposite leg each time.

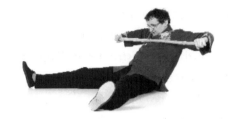

Figure 12.1

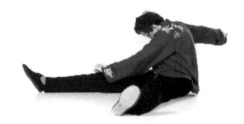

Figure 12.2

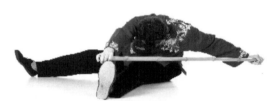

Figure 12.3

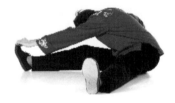

Figure 12.4

STAGE 2 METAL 金 TO FINAL STAGE YANG 阳

Continue in the above method to push the Gan a little further down your left and right legs with each progression until you reach the toes of each foot. Figure 12.3 shows the left side, Figure 12.4 the right side of the Yang stage.

BEGINNING STAGE YIN 阴 TO FINAL STAGE YANG 阳

Miss out the various stages and go from the beginning stage to the final stage, repeating as many times as you are able. At the end of your last repetition, hold your Yin stage position for a count of six.

ADAPTATION

Again, if you find it difficult to get to a 45 degree angle, sit straight and then just go back a few inches as far as you are comfortable (you can still obtain great benefit by doing so).

ENERGY ACTIVATION: ROCKING THE PYRAMID

The twisting and stretching movements of this exercise activate the dual energy centres, constantly moving Qi from the Huiyin point at the base of the spine to the Baihui point at the top of the head. This has a flushing energising effect on the body as the energy is kept in steady motion. You may want to visualise fire or heat rising up your back as you perform the bending twists, then as you return to the beginning Yin position with the Gan on your upper chest, you may imagine Yin cooling water flowing down the front of the body to the Huiyin point. See Figure 12.5.

Notes

This exercise targets the shoulders, arms, neck, chest, entire back, waist, hips, buttocks and of course the legs. It will trim your waistline and firm muscles in your thighs. Set a slow and comfortable pace. If it is difficult to perform this exercise with knees bent, you may find it easier to start off with them only slightly bent as in the example figures in this book. When you are used to the exercise you will be able to bend your knees a little more. 'The Rocking

Bear' is a fantastic exercise for the waist, back and thighs and strengthens the muscles around the hips.

Yin-Yang Energy Activation
Rocking the Pyramid

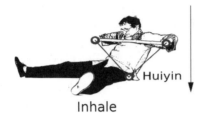

Yin position: feel cooling water flowing down the front of the body to the Huiyin point at the base of the spine

Inhale

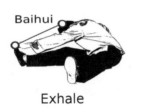

Yang position: feel fire rising up the spine to the Baihui point at the top of the head

Exhale

Figure 12.5

13 Tailor's Walk 裁缝步行

BEGINNING STAGE YIN 阴

Sit on the floor with your legs straight out in front of you with your knees slightly bent. Hold the Gan against the back of your shoulders in a wide grip. Keep your eyes and head facing directly ahead at all times in this exercise. Keep your back relaxed but straight. This exercise has no set breathing, but when you establish a 'walking' rhythm, you should breathe easily in tune with your movements.

Walk Forwards on Your Buttocks

STAGE 1 EARTH 土

Bring your left heel forwards and twist your upper body at the waist to the right, and bring your left elbow forwards slightly.

STAGE 2 METAL 金

Bring your right heel forwards and twist your upper body at the waist, twisting to the left and bringing your right elbow forwards slightly.

STAGE 3 WATER 水

Bring your left heel forwards and twist your upper body at the waist to the right and bring your left elbow forwards a bit further.

STAGE 4 WOOD 木

Bring your right heel forwards and twist your upper body at the waist to the left and bring your right elbow forwards a bit further.

STAGE 5 FIRE 火

Bring your left heel forwards and twist your upper body at the waist to the right, bringing your left elbow forwards so that it is over the left knee.

FINAL STAGE YANG 阳

Bring your right heel forwards and twist your upper body at the waist to the left and bring your right elbow forwards so that it is past the knees, the Gan touching your chin or neck.

Walk Backwards on Your Buttocks

STAGE 1 EARTH 土

Twist at the waist to the right while placing the right heel backwards and bring the right elbow back slightly; simultaneously shift the right hip backwards to move the right buttock back.

STAGE 2 METAL 金

Twist at the waist to the left while placing the left heel backwards and bringing the left elbow back slightly; simultaneously shift the left hip backwards to move the left buttock back.

STAGE 3 WATER 水

Twist at the waist to the right while placing the right heel backwards and bring the right elbow back further; simultaneously shift the right hip backwards to move the right buttock back.

STAGE 4 WOOD 木

Twist at the waist to the left while placing the left heel backwards and bring the left elbow back further; simultaneously shift the left hip backwards to move the left buttock back.

STAGE 5 FIRE 火

Twist at the waist to the right while placing the right heel backwards and bringing the right elbow back further again; simultaneously shift the right hip backwards to move the right buttock back.

FINAL STAGE YANG 阳

Twist at the waist to the left while placing the left heel backwards and bringing the left elbow back as far as you can so the right elbow is past the knees and the Gan touching your chin or neck; simultaneously shift the left hip backwards to move the left buttock back.

BEGINNING STAGE YIN 阴 TO FINAL STAGE YANG 阳 (FORWARDS)

'Walk' forwards on your buttocks, eliminating the stages, five times, making sure your elbows swing as far as possible and that both hands alternately reach the front of your face. Remember that the same side elbows and heels work together; when the left heel moves forwards the left elbow does also; when the right heel moves forwards so does the right elbow. Ensure that your forward arm's hand ends up in front of your face alternately each time you twist backwards.

BEGINNING STAGE YIN 阴 TO FINAL STAGE YANG 阳 (BACKWARDS)

Then 'walk' backwards on your buttocks, eliminating the stages, five times, making sure your elbows swing as far as possible. Remember that the same side elbows and heels work together; when the left heel moves backwards, the left elbow does also; and when the right heel moves backwards so does the right elbow.

Repetition of Forwards-Backwards Sets

Continue to walk forwards five times and backwards five times in the same way as described, as many times as is comfortable for you. Figures 13.1 and 13.2 show the left and right sides of the walk.

ADAPTATION

If you cannot get your elbows over your knees as you walk, swing them as far as you can.

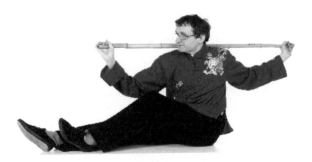

Figure 13.1

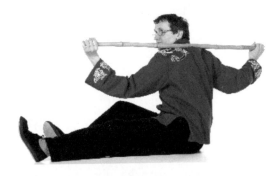

Figure 13.2

ENERGY ACTIVATION: WALKING THE PYRAMID

The twisting and 'walking' movements of this exercise activate the dual energy centres, constantly moving Qi from the Huiyin point at the base of the spine to the Baihui point at the top of the head. You may want to visualise fire or heat rising up your back and Yin cooling water flowing down the front of your body constantly – but the timing of this visualisation is left up to the individual in this exercise. See Figure 13.3.

Notes

'Tailor's Walk' is a complete floor exercise and although you may find it difficult at first, persevere and you will find it becomes easier over the weeks as the muscles in your 'core' region strengthen (see below). This exercise particularly strengthens muscles in the lower back lumber region, loosens the hips and strengthens the muscles around the hips. At the first attempt most people can only perform a few of these 'walking steps' because this exercise targets muscles not used in most activities. Therefore even people who consider themselves fit may be surprised at how few walks they can perform on their first attempt. During this exercise the most common sensation is one of becoming warm, because the twisting of your upper body and stretching greatly improves blood circulation.

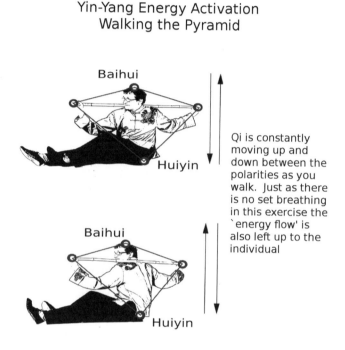

Yin-Yang Energy Activation
Walking the Pyramid

Qi is constantly moving up and down between the polarities as you walk. Just as there is no set breathing in this exercise the `energy flow' is also left up to the individual

Figure 13.3

Core Muscles

The floor exercises are all effective in developing the body's 'core muscles'. Core strength comes from muscles that are less obvious and visible than many muscles and their development enables you to stay fit well into old age, to stand straighter and have more energy than your peers. The core muscles include not only those in your abdominals and back, but also muscles in your pelvic floor and hips. Many of your core muscles cannot be seen because they are buried underneath other muscles. For example:

- The transverse abdominis keeps your posture upright and protects many of your internal organs.

- The erector spinae behind the body supports the back.
- Pelvic floor muscles aid in stabilising the spine.

All these muscles, and more, work together to keep the trunk stable while the limbs are active. Strong core muscles keep your back healthy, hold your body upright and improve your balance. If the core muscles are weak, your body does not work as effectively and other muscles have to pick up the 'slack'. This can result in injuries such as a twisted knee, a pulled shoulder or bad back. A weak core can make you old before your time, but with a strong core you may be old in years but you won't walk old.

14 Rolling the Panda 熊猫辗压

BEGINNING STAGE YIN 阴

Sit on the floor with your knees bent, heels together. Place the Gan over your ankles, lifting your toes up to prevent it rolling off. Place your hands between your knees and thread them underneath, right hand under right knee and left hand under left knee, so that they come out around the outside of your ankles, and grasp the Gan, palms up, knuckles towards the floor (Figure 14.1). Important: keep your heels together, your back and shoulders rounded at all times and your chin tucked into your neck all through this exercise. This exercise is done in *two phases*: beginner's and advanced. Usually, Phase One (the beginner's phase) should be practised for some weeks before attempting Phase Two (the advanced phase).

Phase One (Beginners)

STAGE 1

Inhale deeply as you rock backwards from the beginning stage very slightly and lift your heels a few inches off the floor (Figure 14.2). Then exhale completely as you roll forwards back to the beginning stage.

STAGE 2

Inhale deeply as you rock backwards a bit further, lifting your heels a bit higher so that your tail bone touches the floor (Figure 14.3). Then exhale completely as you roll forwards back to the beginning stage.

STAGE 3

Inhale deeply as you rock right back, keeping the body locked in this rounded position, so that your back is on the floor and you are looking at the ceiling or sky (Figure 14.4). Then, using your momentum, immediately exhale completely sas you roll forwards, back to the beginning stage.

Go from the beginning to final stage for several repetitions, smoothly. After a few days or weeks – which varies with the individual – you will be ready to move on to the advanced phase.

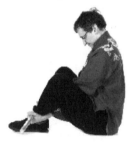

Figure 14.1

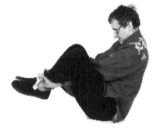

Figure 14.2

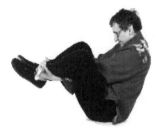

Figure 14.3

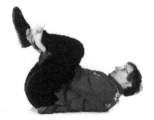

Figure 14.4

Phase Two (Advanced)

You begin the exercise by going through Phase One first. Then you do the following.

STAGE 1

From the beginning position, inhale deeply as you rock backwards, under control, so that your shoulders are some inches off the floor (Figure 14.5). Then exhale completely as you roll forwards, back to the beginning stage. Perform this sequence as many times as you are able. After a few days or weeks – which varies with the individual – you will be ready to move to Stage 2 of the advanced phase. Again you must begin the exercise by going through Phase One a few times first, then go through Stage 1 of the advanced phase a few times also before doing the following.

STAGE 2

Inhale deeply as you rock backwards, under control, so that your middle back is touching the floor. Then exhale completely as you slowly roll forwards to the beginning stage. Perform this sequence as many times as you are able. After a few days or weeks – which varies with the individual – you will be ready to move to the final, most difficult stage. Again you must begin the exercise by going through Phase One first and then the advanced Stages 1 and 2 a few times before doing the following.

STAGE 3: FINAL STAGE

Inhale deeply as you rock back, under control, so that only your lower back is touching the floor (Figure 14.6). Then exhale completely as you slowly roll forwards to the beginning stage. Repeat this as many times as you are able. After the advanced stage has been mastered, you start the exercise each time by going through Phase One, then the advanced phase (Stages 1 and 2) again in the way described.

Figure 14.7 shows Phase One, Stage 3.

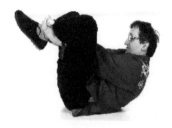

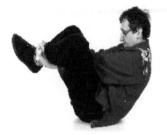

Figure 14.5   Figure 14.6

Phase One (Stage 3)

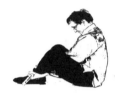

Inhale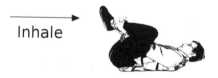

Exhale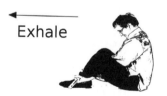

Figure 14.7

ADAPTATION

This is a difficult exercise and many people will not be able to go to the positions as directed. Nevertheless those who do not or cannot go onto their backs should just do the first part (lifting the feet a few inches from the floor). A little exercise is better than none. As for those who cannot even lift their feet, they should be able to 'assume the position' and do the breathing, 'trying' to lift their feet, which will exercise the same muscles as if they could actually lift their feet. On no account should this exercise be missed out simply because you cannot lift your feet from the ground.

ENERGY ACTIVATION: ROLLING THE PYRAMID

In this exercise, Qi is kept locked by your position and the rocking movement activates the dual energy centres, constantly moving Qi from the Huiyin point at the base of the spine to the Baihui point at the top of the head. The pyramid formed by the hands is a much narrower one than in most of the exercises. You may want to visualise Yin cooling water flowing down the front of the body to the Huiyin point when moving backwards, then when moving forwards you may imagine fire or heat rising up your back. See Figure 14.8.

Notes

Because of the ingenious position of the body and placing of the Gan, your back is protected from any injury or strain during this exercise. It is the abdominal and stomach muscles that move the body, not the back. Although the back does get exercised, it is protected as it is gently massaged when we roll on and off it using a suitable surface such as an exercise mat. Perseverance in the exercise will bring you absolute evidence that your lower abdominals are getting stronger because the only way you can perform the later stages is by preparing your muscles by going through the first and second stages first. Gentle perseverance brings reward. This exercise also works the neck, shoulders, chest, waist, hips, buttocks and legs, and works wonders on flattening the stomach.

Yin-Yang Energy Activation
Rolling the Pyramid

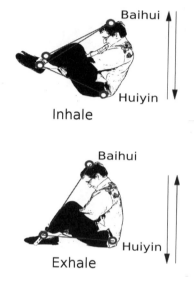

Qi constantly flows from the Baihui point at the top of the head to the Huiyin point at the base of the spine; the sequence of activation is left up to the individual. You may feel raising energy either while coming forwards or going backwards

Figure 14.8

15 Raising the Bird's Wing 鸟翼上升

Right Side

Go through every stage lying on your right side.

BEGINNING STAGE YIN 阴

Lie on your right side and place the Gan vertically next to you at arm's length as if you are holding a flag pole, your right hand grasping the base and your left hand about halfway up. Keep your body in a straight line and your legs straight out, left leg on top of the right. Do not let your head drop to the floor during this exercise and keep knees locked and toes pointed at all times (Figure 15.1).

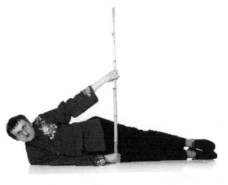

Figure 15.1

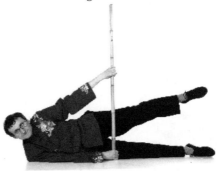

Figure 15.2

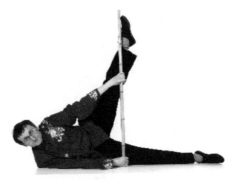

Figure 15.3

STAGE 1 EARTH 土

Inhale deeply as you raise your left leg about ten inches above your right leg. Then exhale completely as you slowly lower your left leg to the starting stage.

STAGE 2 METAL 金

Inhale deeply as you raise your left leg a little further than Stage 1 in the same way (Figure 15.2). Then exhale completely as you slowly lower your left leg to the starting stage.

STAGE 3 WATER 水 TO STAGE 5 FIRE 火

Inhale deeply as you raise your left leg a little further each time. Then exhale completely as you slowly lower your left leg to the starting stage.

FINAL STAGE YANG 阳

Inhale deeply as you raise your left leg until you touch your toes against the top of the Gan. Hold this position for two seconds (Figure 15.3). Then exhale completely as you slowly lower your left leg to the starting stage.

BEGINNING STAGE YIN 阴 TO FINAL STAGE YANG 阳

Repeat as many times as you are able, slowly lifting your left leg to the top of the Gan and slowly lowering it in the way described, eliminating the intermediate stages; each time you touch your toes against the Gan, you hold for two seconds.

Left Side

Now repeat the whole exercise by lying on your left side and going through all the stages with your right leg raised.

ENERGY ACTIVATION: RAISING THE PYRAMID

In this exercise you create a double pyramid. The first pyramid is made by your hands as you hold the Gan in position and this maintains Qi. You create the second pyramid as you raise your legs, which activates Qi. You may want to visualise fire or heat rising up your back and Yin cooling water flowing down the front of the body when you either raise or lower your legs – it is up to individuals how they interpret the energy flow in this exercise. See Figure 15.4.

Yin-Yang Energy Activation
Raising the Pyramid

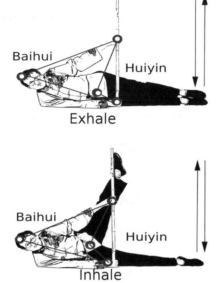

Qi constantly flows from the Baihui point at the top of the head to the Huiyin point at the base of the spine; the sequence of activation is left up to the individual. You may feel rising energy either while raising or lowering your legs

Figure 15.4

ADAPTATION

This is one of the simplest exercises to adapt. Simply raise your legs as far as they will go. It does not matter that they cannot reach the top of the Gan, but you should go as far as possible without straining.

Notes

Pay attention to the Golden Ratio breathing so that your legs descend more slowly than when they are raised. This exercise is excellent not only for the legs but also for the waist, hips, buttocks and the entire back. The upper body also receives a workout as you hold your head up from the floor and hold the Gan in position. The raised leg must remain in contact with the Gan at all times.

16 Dragon Kicks 龙腿上升

BEGINNING STAGE YIN 阴

Lie on the floor, on your stomach, and grasp the Gan with both hands close together in the centre of the Gan, knuckles faced upwards and elbows about a 45 degree angle from the Gan (Figure 16.1). During this exercise try to hold up your head and chin as far as is comfortable. Keep your legs straight (knees locked) and toes pointed at all times during this exercise.

Right Leg

Go through every stage raising your right leg.

STAGE 1 EARTH 土

Inhale deeply as you raise your right leg a few inches off the floor. Then exhale completely as you slowly lower your right leg to the starting stage.

STAGE 2 METAL 金

Inhale deeply as you raise your right leg again, this time a few more inches off the floor (Figure 16.2). Then exhale completely as you slowly lower your right leg to the starting stage.

STAGE 3 WATER 水 TO FINAL STAGE YANG 阳

Inhale deeply as you raise your right leg a little further each time, until it reaches the final stage, where it will be as high as you are able to lift it (Figure 16.3). Then exhale completely as you slowly lower your right leg to the starting stage.

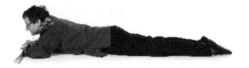

Figure 16.1

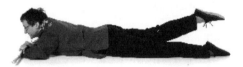

Figure 16.2

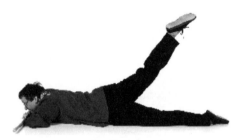

Figure 16.3

BEGINNING STAGE YIN 阴 TO FINAL STAGE YANG 阳

Repeat as many times as you are able, lifting your right leg in the way described, eliminating the in-between stages. It is impossible to estimate the final Yang stage so simply raise your leg a little higher each stage until you reach your natural 'Yang' – that is, as far as you can comfortably reach after the five stages. Then during your final repetitions see if you can lift your leg a little higher each time.

On the final repetition, hold the Yang position for a count of two, then very slowly lower your leg to the beginning position.

Left Leg

Now repeat the whole exercise by going through all the stages but this time raising your left leg.

ADAPTATIONS

The 'Inch-by-Inch' method is essential for *everyone* in this exercise. You will then find that your final, Yang position gives you freedom to extend your legs further upward with each repetition, should you be able to do so.

ENERGY ACTIVATION: KICKING THE PYRAMID

This exercise is similar to the previous one as you create a double pyramid. The first pyramid is made by your hands as you hold the Gan in position, and this maintains Qi. You create the second pyramid as you raise your legs, which activates Qi. You may want to visualise fire or heat rising up your back and Yin cooling water flowing down the front of the body when you either raise or lower your legs – it is up to individuals how they interpret the energy flow in this exercise. See Figure 16.4.

Yin-Yang Energy Activation
Kicking the Pyramid

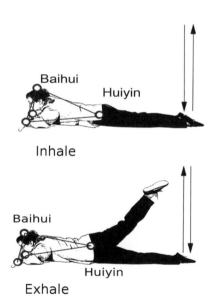

Baihui

Huiyin

Inhale

Baihui

Huiyin

Exhale

Qi constantly flows from the Baihui point at the top of the head to the Huiyin point at the base of the spine; the sequence of activation is left up to the individual. You may feel rising energy either while raising or lowering your legs

Figure 16.4

Notes

Do not underestimate the effectiveness of this exercise. Perform it in a relaxed manner led by Golden Ratio breathing. Leave yourself plenty of room and never strain or force your leg further than is comfortable. Even a few inches of progress performing the five graduated stages is better than nothing. Make sure you slowly lower your leg each time, with the exhalation, which massages and gently stretches the muscles of the back as well as loosens the hips. The leg on the ground actually does a lot of work. Be constantly aware during this exercise that you are performing an internal, gentle art. Relax and move well within your means at all times. As with the previous exercise, be especially aware of the breathing leading the movements and allow the Golden Ratio breathing cycle to work its 'magic', ensuring that your legs descend more slowly than they are raised.

17 Shoulder Shrugs 聳肩

BEGINNING STAGE

Stand straight, feet in a close stance, and place the Gan behind you, grasping it at shoulder width, knuckles forwards (Figure 17.1). Look directly ahead and keep your chin up, arms straight by your sides, elbows locked.

STAGE 1

Inhale deeply as you raise your shoulders up as high as you can, trying to touch your ears (Figure 17.2). Then throw your shoulders back as far as you can (Figure 17.3). Make sure your arms remain straight, elbows locked as you do so. Hold your breath.

STAGE 2

Exhale completely as you lower your shoulders very slightly as you move your shoulders forwards (Figure 17.4).

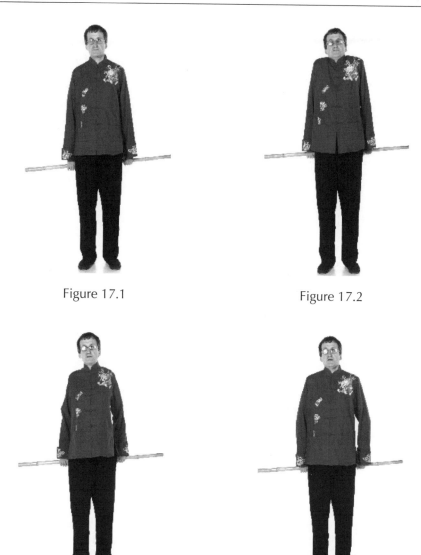

Figure 17.1

Figure 17.2

Figure 17.3

Figure 17.4

REPETITIONS

Repeat at least eight times, ensuring that the Gan remains in contact with your body, with your back straight and arms locked.

ENERGY ACTIVATION: SHRUGGING THE PYRAMID

In this exercise you not only raise and lower the pyramid and Qi but also 'lock in' Qi at the same time. The idea of this exercise is that it helps you store and maintain Qi accumulated and activated in all the previous exercises. You can visualise cooling Yin energy flowing down the front of your body while inhaling and moving your shoulders up and back, then visualise Yang fire energy rising up your spine when exhaling and moving your shoulders forwards. See Figure 17.5.

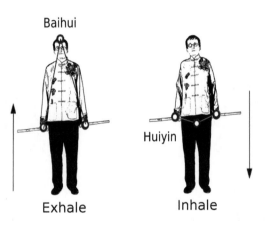

Yin-Yang Energy Activation
Shrugging the Pyramid

Baihui

Huiyin

Exhale

Inhale

Although this is the 'Yin' position, the pyramid is focused upwards; feel fire rising up the spine to the Baihui point at the top of the head

Although this is the 'Yang' position, the pyramid is focused downwards; feel cooling water flowing down the front of the body to the Huiyin point at the base of the spine

Figure 17.5

Notes

This exercise is one of the best possible for developing good posture. Its importance in the Jiangan 17 Exercises Routine is that it allows your body to 'lock in' energy you have produced during all the previous exercises. The shrugs work on your upper body only and involve the neck, shoulders, chest and arms. Your shoulders do all the work and are not assisted by your arms. You will notice that this is also a good exercise to tighten and firm abdominal muscles.

8

Variations and Advanced Exercises

THE SPECIAL BEGINNER'S ROUTINE: LESS IS MORE

When I began teaching Jiangan, I was surprised by the number of young, supposedly fit and able-bodied people who were unable to manoeuvre the Gan past the first few stages of each exercise. There are also many elderly and frail people who will be unable to move past the first positions. The inability to perform the 'ideal' Yang stages may discourage some people, who may think that the exercises are too difficult and give up practice altogether. Students should regard the Yang stages shown in this book as future points on a journey and should not perform the advanced stages until they are ready and able to do so. Here I must mention a humorous but exasperating trait of human nature that manifests in most exercise classes. I have observed, as a teacher, that the eye is stronger than the ear. Students tend to copy what the teacher does rather than what they are told to do. Within a group of students watching their instructor performing an advanced posture (and told that *on no account must they copy*), invariably one or two will try. So I have developed a very rudimentary adaptation of the exercises in this book consisting of two phases that are practised with a simple and beneficial breathing method (a pattern to familiarise the beginner with Golden Ratio breathing). In the first phase the student simply holds the Gan in the beginning Yin position, *inhaling for three seconds and exhaling for five seconds.* This timing is not absolute but serves as a guide; later students can lengthen the breaths as long as they maintain a ratio of about 3:5. After all 17 Exercises have been practised in this manner comfortably and smoothly, students may then practise the second phase. This consists of merely performing the first (earth) stage of each exercise as outlined in the main instructions but using the Golden Ratio 3:5 seconds inhalation to exhalation. When individuals feel comfortable with this second phase they can move on to the 'Inch-by-Inch' method outlined in the next section until they reach their natural Yang position.

This special beginner's form ensures that students receive a sense of completion even if they do not reach the ideal Yang positions. It is also a great leveller; everyone in the class performs similar movements no matter what their physical ability. In the long run it does not matter if a student reaches only the first phase of the beginner's routine because he or she is still getting great benefit from the movements, breathing, meditation and body alignment. It also keeps the holistic value of performing all the exercises in the correct sequence. It is most important that those unable to reach the ideal Yang positions in any of the exercises do *not* cut out the exercise completely but adapt it by only going as far as they are able. Even 'assuming the position' of a beginning posture, making the effort to move correctly and using correct breathing is very beneficial.

INCH-BY-INCH METHOD

Carrying on from the special beginner's routine, the 'Inch-by-Inch' method is another useful way to ensure that weak, infirm and elderly people can get maximum benefit without straining their bodies. It is similar to the special beginner's routine but you advance a little further – in stages of about an inch or so with each breathing cycle, until your own limit is reached. Again, even if the final Yang position corresponds to a fit young person's 'first' or 'second' stage, it does not matter: it will still provide great benefit because the movements target the same muscle groups and body parts as the advanced positions.

MULTI-STAGES METHOD

Splitting the exercises into five graduated stages based on the Five Elements is the most convenient division of the exercises, but it is possible to divide them into more stages if you wish. Focusing on the intermediate stages rather than the Yin-Yang repetitions can be particularly advantageous for those who find the Yang stages challenging. Anyone who adopts this approach will get as much benefit from the exercises as those able to go to the extreme positions. The 'multi-stage' method can also be used by anyone to put in a light extra practice session in the middle of the day or while at work, and at these times there is no need to progress to the Yang position. Jiangan is adaptable to individual lifestyles but there must be no compromise on the *minimum* number of stages; at least five stages must be used if you are proceeding to your own Yang position. If you try to skip these stages or perform less – particularly with jerky bouncy movements – you risk straining yourself and will not get real benefit from the system. It is not only the movements but also the method that gives the system its unique potency. However, the minimum of five stages does not apply to the special beginner's routine or 'Inch-by-Inch' method.

ADVANCED EXERCISES

The 17 Exercises Routine is adequate for developing abundant health and well-being for everyone. However, I also practise several additional exercises that I witnessed in Malaysia and reconstructed from my rudimentary drawings. In fact, there are hundreds of Jiangan exercises but the majority are just variations or versions of the 17 Exercises Routine. The exercises described in this chapter must be attempted only if you can comfortably perform the Yang stages as suggested in Chapter 7. Furthermore, you should attempt these advanced exercises only when you have been practising Jiangan regularly for many months, perhaps a year or so. Even then, ensure that you first go through the 17 Exercises Routine and do not attempt to substitute these advanced exercises for them. These additional exercises are for people who require a further degree of suppleness and fitness. I must stress that despite being interesting and very rewarding, the advanced exercises are not essential for everyday health and fitness for the average person. They can be performed either during the 17 Exercises Routine (making it longer) or after the standard routine has been completed.

Twisting the Snake with Left and Right Turn

This is one of the easier variations and most people should be able to perform it to a certain degree. It is exactly like the 'Twisting the Snake' exercise but as you inhale deeply and move your right hand to the left over the side of your head, you also turn your upper body to the left; then you turn your upper body back to the front when the Gan is behind your body. In the second part of the exercise when you exhale and move your left arm over your head to the right, also turn your upper body to the right then return to face the front as you come back to the beginning posture. Repeat the process with your left arm leading; turning first to the right then to the left as you return to the beginning position. This exercise can be performed immediately after the normal 'Twisting the Snake'. In this case you do not have to go through five graduated stages but merely perform the Yang stage.

Twisting the Snake Spirals

This is the only advanced exercise that is not based on any of the 17 Exercises Routine. With feet in a wide position, begin with the Gan behind your back in the Yang position of the 'Peeling the Octopus' and 'Twisting the Snake' exercises (the Gan resting against the buttocks between thumb and forefinger). Inhale deeply. Then exhale while turning to the left, simultaneously raising your right arm over your head to the left then down in front of your body (the right fist along your centre), and bend your upper body and turn to the right while following your right fist with your eyes as it moves across the body at the height of your thighs. You are moving in an anti-clockwise direction. When your left fist reaches the front of your body, transfer focus to this hand, following it to the right; inhale deeply when your left hand is approximately above your right foot, then follow it up to head height, in front of and close to your body, where it moves back and around your head to the left, coming to rest with the Gan back in the rear Yang position again, resting against the buttocks. Now you repeat this exercise in the opposite, clockwise, direction, leading with your left hand as you exhale and turn to the right. In this very exhilarating exercise you can imagine a vertical clock face in front of your body. The focus should be at '6 o'clock' (where the hand–eye focus changes) and '12 o'clock' (where the arms cross over the head). This exercise must be performed in the usual five stages, beginning at thigh height and ending at the ankles. Your legs must be straight, knees locked and facing forwards at all times, and only your upper body turning.

Twitching the Dragon's Tail (Slanted Combination)

This is a variation that is strictly for the advanced practitioner, as it combines the twist and bend from 'Twitching the Dragon's Tail' *in one movement*. From the beginning posture, inhale deeply. Then as you exhale fully, bend a little to the left while also moving your left hand a little to the right, which produces a slanting effect. Do the same on the right side until you get to your personal Yang position. Young, fit and able-bodied people should end up looking directly to the front but with their leading elbow just in front of their groin. This variation twists the upper body considerably so care must be taken to use as many stages as you require and to work well within yourself.

Twitching the Dragon's Tail (Twists) Combined with The Tiger Springs

This is a challenging and difficult exercise that demands a great deal of coordination and suppleness. It must not be attempted unless you are advanced. Only the Yang sequence will be described here but the experienced practitioner can work out the various stages. It consists of The Tiger Springs with the Gan over the back of your shoulders, but with each lunge (ensuring that you lean back so that your weight remains equally on both legs), twist the opposite arm to the leading leg forwards until the Yang stage, where your rear knee will be on the floor and your leading hand ends up in front of your face as in the twists of the 'Twitching the Dragon's Tail' exercise.

Twisting the Snake Combined with The Tiger Springs

This is another difficult exercise but very rewarding. It increases flexibility and has beneficial effects on the entire back region. Again only the Yang sequence will be described here but the experienced practitioner can work out the various stages. From the beginning posture of 'Twisting the Snake', inhale deeply. Then as you exhale fully, bring your right arm around your left side, turning to the left with your upper body. Then as you turn back to face the front, step forwards with your right leg so that your left knee is on the ground; by this time the Gan is behind your body close to the Yang position of the 'Peeling the Octopus' and 'Twisting the Snake' posture – but instead of resting against your buttocks, the Gan is pushed out a few inches away from your body, elbows locked. Make sure you lean backwards so that your weight is distributed on both legs equally. Do not put all your weight on your front leg. In the second part of the exercise, inhale deeply as you turn to the right and bring your left arm around the right side of your body and move back rapidly to the beginning standing position as the Gan returns to its position in front of your body. Now repeat this with your left leg forwards and leading with the left arm. You can also perform this exercise leading with the opposite arm to the stepping leg (right arm lead, left leg forwards and vice versa).

Side Thrust Tiger Springs

This is similar to the original 'The Tiger Springs'; the footwork is the same and again you lean back to ensure that the leading foot that steps out does not take all the weight. From the beginning posture, step forwards on your right foot and thrust the Gan to the right, horizontally at shoulder height, while also turning your upper body to the right. When you have performed the five stages, step forwards with your left foot and thrust the Gan out to the left in the same way. You can also perform this exercise by alternating arms and legs so that you turn and thrust out to the opposite side to the leading foot.

Horse Stance on a Tightrope Variations

The first three exercises ('Sunrise and Sunset', 'Peeling the Octopus' and 'Twisting the Snake') can be performed while in the 'Horse Stance on a Tightrope' posture, going from straight locked knees position into a semi-squat, but with some changes:

- Do not go up onto your toes in 'Sunrise and Sunset', but keep the original breathing method.

- Add the sinking movement to 'Peeling the Octopus', while keeping the original breathing method.

- In the 'Twisting the Snake' exercise, inhale and sink as you move the Gan behind your body, then exhale and rise up to return to the beginning position standing with straight legs and locked knees again.

The graduated stages should be used for these variations.

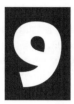

Health Benefits

Although there has not been the opportunity to conduct medical studies on Jiangan, there is much anecdotal evidence to show that it is as effective as other Eastern exercise systems in improving health, especially in the areas in which they have been medically tested. The full range of Jiangan's efficiency is difficult to estimate, but I am certain that the following list is not definitive:

- Alleviating psychological disorders and easing stress.

- Alleviating chronic breathing ailments.

- Improving strength and muscle tone.

- Improving cardiovascular fitness.

- Reducing osteoarthritis pain.

- Improving flexibility and balance.

- Lowering and regulating blood pressure.

- Promoting good digestion.

- Reducing falls in elderly people.

- Improving blood flow in injured muscles and joints.

Bruce Johnson observed that every exercise in the system had outstanding beneficial qualities and that taken as a whole, the entire 17 Exercises Routine is effective at treating many long-standing medical problems. For example, even the most basic and simple movement of holding the Gan in a wide grip and pushing it up and stretching loosens the shoulders and raises the ribcage, which improves its elasticity to help improve lung capacity. The primary reason for performing Jiangan slowly and gently while using the particular twisting, stretching and turning of the upper body is essentially for the benefit of the Five Internal Organs – the heart, liver, lungs, kidneys and spleen – which are extremely important in traditional Chinese medicine. Jiangan gently massages and stimulates them.

HEALTH VERSUS FITNESS?

The major difference between Jiangan and other Eastern health systems is its ability to affect the external shape of the body to a significant degree. It is often said that 'internal' and 'external' exercises are as different as night and day. But the reality is not so clear cut. Although the internal arts have many health benefits, I know from personal experience that it is possible to practise them and still not be in top physical shape. When I began studying Jiangan, I had been practising Taiji for many years. Spending most of my working life sitting at a desk, Taiji certainly helped keep me active, avoid repetitive strain injury and prevent posture problems arising from sitting at a keyboard. But like many men of my age, I had accumulated a modest middle-aged spread, a sign that the body is not in optimum condition. One month after I began practising Jiangan, the muscles in my middle and lower back were firmer and my knees felt much stronger. Several weeks later I was so much trimmer and leaner that friends asked if I had been training in a gym. My 'core' muscles were strengthened considerably, particularly by the floor exercises, and this enhanced my Taiji practice beyond measure. I could perform one leg stances with more confidence and less effort and squat more easily because my legs were strengthened and hip flexibility improved. Whenever I kneel these days, I can feel my calf muscles stronger and firmer than they ever were. While it can be argued that similar body-shaping results can be obtained from industrious workouts in other more robust types of exercise, the fact remains that it was Jiangan, the gentle internal art, that worked – and did so while I kept my lifestyle largely unchanged.

It is clear that you can regularly practise Eastern internal health systems and still be 'out of condition' and accumulate unwanted pounds. The oft heard assertion that you can be overweight and still 'healthy' is emotionally and intellectually unconvincing and should be put into the perspective of the natural world. If you took an overweight cat or dog to a vet, the animal would be declared *unhealthy*. In humans, obesity in developed countries is a huge problem and can be the prime cause of medical problems such as lower back pain, bad circulation, stress and high blood pressure. If we are promoting 'health', we must tackle one of the major health risks in the modern world and so the active promotion of weight loss must be high on the agenda of any health system. Being overweight makes you prone to circulation problems, stress and high blood pressure, and while Eastern internal arts are effective at tackling these symptoms, one could make the point that if people were fitter and trimmer these symptoms might not be such a problem. Although internal arts stress the inner body, they should not neglect the outer body. In fact, the outer body is a reflection of the inner. We know that our skin complexion, for example, deteriorates as a result of what we consume internally such as fatty food, tobacco, alcohol and drugs. Being overweight is no different; it is a symptom of an unhealthy lifestyle. Daily practice of Jiangan helps to tackle the 'external' problems of the body as well as the internal.

How is it that Jiangan can encourage weight loss and fat reduction more effectively? The major premise of this book is that Jiangan was developed to deal with the problem of sedentary lifestyle in the Imperial family and so the exercises include *slightly* more robust and targeted stretches, providing a good cardiovascular workout for those who need it and toning muscles extremely effectively while keeping within the 'gentle exercise mode'. Anyone who doubts the liberating effect of losing excess weight and strengthening and toning essential muscles will experience a pleasant surprise after a few weeks of daily Jiangan practice. You will walk with easier, lighter steps, feel more nimble and agile, have more energy and your quality of life will improve immeasurably. Not only will you experience the benefits you would undoubtedly have obtained from Yoga, Qigong or Taiji but also you will enjoy more tangible physical improvements that will help you in your everyday tasks.

SEDENTARY LIFESTYLE

People in modern industrialised societies have very much the same health issues as rulers in the ancient world, who ate as much rich food as they liked, had access to the finest wines of the time and did not have to work to survive. Many were carried everywhere in sedans. Just as these 'captive animals' of China were given back their life balance with Jiangan, people in the modern world can avail themselves of this magnificent system. I was a civil servant for 18 years and so know the potential problems of sitting at a desk looking at a computer screen for most of the day. Again the lifestyle of the Chinese Imperial family is a vivid parallel with modern-day office workers. While we may have swapped sedan chairs and thrones for swivel chairs and desks, we are essentially the same humans with the same sedentary lifestyle problem. Jiangan is effective and therapeutic for 'office conditions' such as repetitive strain injury, lower back pain and other problems caused by sitting for long periods at a keyboard. The standing exercises in particular will work wonders for the shoulders, arms, hands, wrists and posture problems. Holding the Gan in a gentle fist 'tasks' and exercises the hands without tiring them. The postures requiring the hands to change position such as 'Peeling the Octopus' and 'Twisting the Snake' are also beneficial to the hands, wrists and fingers.

Obesity

Jiangan is an extremely suitable exercise for overweight people and even the morbidly obese can benefit greatly from its unique methodology and low-impact nature. Obesity is more than having a few extra pounds. It is having an accumulation of fat in your body that increases your risk of heart disease and diabetes and knocks years off your life. In the UK obesity has trebled since 1980 as our lifestyles have changed; increased consumption of convenience foods and 'school run culture' have seen obesity in children in particular rise at an alarming rate in recent years. Particularly advantageous for large people is Jiangan's methodology for postures; weight is *never* placed mainly on one leg, which puts pressure on the knees. As well as improving flexibility, circulation and balance, the exercises tone and stretch muscles gradually and safely so that they are able to bear weight more easily. The cardiovascular element also encourages weight loss and so it is possible to burn calories with Jiangan. It is this extra element – the ability to become slightly more robust and expend a little more exertion but still remain in the internal framework – which gave Jiangan its weight-reducing reputation in the USA when it was promoted by Bruce Johnson. The genius of the floor exercises in particular is that they can really trim the waist, lower abdominals and thighs almost as effectively as gym machines but without exhaustion or making the heart pump too fast.

With all this emphasis on losing weight and toning muscle, it is important not to focus too much on 'body image'. Eastern heath systems work on the internal system, which is more effective and healthy than simply building muscles or a shapely body for its own sake. But external appearance reflects inner health and lifestyle and so must not be ignored either.

Restoring Male and Female Body Shapes

Jiangan aims at restoring the natural balance of the body and lifestyle. Evolution has produced a typical universal body type for men and women. If we look at people in developing countries, their shape still reflects the natural 'optimum norm' that industrialised countries have lost in recent decades. The classical shape for men is slim and wiry, which helps them perform active tasks such as running, fighting and hunting. The classical shape for women is for them to have a little more body fat which is conducive to child-bearing. This is not a judgemental statement on the roles of the sexes but merely an observation on the optimum state that nature has determined for humans over thousands of years. Industrialised nations have got the balance wrong; women are encouraged to be thin stick insects and men are encouraged to turn themselves into muscular 'hunks' and build up bulk. Daily practice of Jiangan helps restore the natural balance of male and female bodies as bodies develop in different ways according to gender. Women need not worry; Jiangan does not build big powerful muscles but makes muscles stronger within the body shape of the individual.

STRAINS, INJURIES AND ALIGNMENT

Performing the 17 Exercises Routine correctly, we engage in a range of beneficial and correct joint, postural and structural alignments. One area where Jiangan has been observed to help in particular is combating a range of back problems. Many people spend their lives in postures that round their back like a turtle. They sit round-shouldered and round-backed, a posture that shortens the chest and shoulder muscles in the front and overstretches and weakens them at the back. Chronically slouching forwards also pushes the discs of the back out. This condition, 'herniation', can press on nearby nerves, sending pain down the back of the leg (sciatica) or arm. Jiangan, particularly the first few postures of the 17 Exercises Routine, can help by opening the chest and shoulder muscles so that posture is improved and muscles become stronger and no longer out of balance.

Jiangan is supreme in treating neck, shoulder and back injuries and many types of strains. If you wake after sleeping awkwardly with pain or stiffness in the shoulder and neck, the pain usually goes after practising the 17 Exercises Routine. Jiangan also strengthens rarely used muscles so that occasional or irregular physical activity such as walking further than you are accustomed to is not such a trauma on the body. For several years, every summer for about a week or so, I look after a house a few miles out in the suburbs. I like to walk into town each morning but the first day of my stay is a shock to my system; my legs, feet and thighs are usually sore. But the first time I made this journey after practising Jiangan for several months, I had absolutely no soreness in any part of my body. Carrying a bag in each hand while wearing a full knapsack can sometimes strain the back. When this has happened to me, the symptoms have disappeared shortly after practising the 17 Exercises Routine. On two occasions when waking with lower back pain caused by over-exertion the previous day, the pain totally disappeared after I performed the 17 Exercises Routine. Clearly there is some special quality about performing the *entire* 17 Exercises Routine in the correct sequence that has a remarkable effect on the body. It is a moving medicine.

The essential point to remember about using Jiangan to treat strains and injuries is never to practise only the exercise targeting the part of the body you presume will benefit. For example if you have a back problem, even floor exercises such as 'Dragon Kicks', if performed correctly, are very potent methods of massaging the muscles of the entire back. It is the combined effect of all the exercises practised in specific order that produces results; the whole is greater than the sum of its parts.

RESPIRATORY DISORDERS

Jiangan can produce significant improvement for sufferers of respiratory disorders in particular. Ever since I was a child I have suffered, during winter months, with chronic and acute Upper Airway Cough Syndrome (UACS) which causes the distressing and debilitating 'post-nasal drip' symptom. Up until recently the attacks were so extreme and debilitating on occasions that I frequently found myself gagging and attempting to vomit the mucus that blocked my airways. Attacks usually lasted several hours or sometimes all day. Although I have been practising Taiji and Qigong routines for over 30 years, during the days of these attacks, my morning sessions have made little impact on my symptoms. But the first winter after practising Jiangan each day, I had only three brief attacks, and on each occasion these disappeared after performing my Jiangan routine. The second winter I was virtually free from UACS and experienced only occasional and mild catarrh.

It is probable that the following factors in Jiangan enhance breathing function and ensure rapid and significant relief for sufferers of repository disorders:

- The wide grip opens the chest muscles and improves the working of the lungs.

- Golden Ratio inhalation-exhalation diaphragmatic breathing is effective because it is the natural breathing pattern employed while we are sleeping or relaxed.

- The stages of each exercise gradually require more oxygen and the breathing becomes deeper as we progress.

INCREASED CIRCULATION AND REGULATION OF BLOOD PRESSURE

Jiangan elicits a cardiovascular response associated with moderate intensity exercise. It can lower and regulate blood pressure. The slow movements combined with deep breathing also make it a superb exercise for elderly people. Unlike robust physical exercises that make the heart pump faster, there is increased circulation from the gentle rhythmic motion of the body combined with deep breathing which works on the veins and arteries and regulates the blood flow throughout the body.

Qi and Healing

Jiangan is not just a physical exercise. Because it is an internal system, the health promoting qualities are enhanced by correct mental focus which can manifest in many ways and are largely up to the ingenuity of the individual. While Chinese philosophical concepts can be rather vague, 'energy work' can be rationalised in terms that are easily understood. Physiologically speaking, the slow movements distribute energy flows or Qi, blood and essential fluids around the body and maintain Yin-Yang balance within the body. Unfortunately, phrases such as 'balance your Qi' or 'balancing your Yin-Yang' are almost compulsory material these days for comedians attacking new age concepts and ideas. But from the standpoint of Chinese internal medicine, intention moves the Qi and Qi moves the blood. Where blood goes, circulation is improved. For some people the notion of Qi may seem fanciful but whether or not Qi exists is a matter of psychology. I do not think Qi has the same level of existence as gravity or electricity or phenomena that can be measured and quantified by the scientific method, but in terms of psychology – or more accurately, metaphysics – everything 'exists'. In fact, it is impossible for anything *not* to exist. Even something conjured in the imagination of an individual or that can be envisaged or dreamed about 'exists' and this is a truism of philosophy. Consequently when we argue about the existence of anything, it is the precise nature of the existence we are disputing. If many rational people were asked whether 'healing energy' exists, they would probably reply in the negative because no scientific tests have ever shown the existence of such a force or indeed how it could possibly operate. Yet the power of visualisation, meditation and focus can achieve certain feats that can be attributed to a 'force' or 'energy' and perhaps we are merely discussing semantics.

My own experience of what could be called healing energy convinced me that the mind is capable of significant input into the working of the physical body. As a child I had warts covering both hands but by my mid-twenties I had only the one on the fourth finger of my left hand. Out of curiosity I decided to test 'Reverse Energy Flow', a healing method taught to me by my teacher. This method consists of visualising the injured part of the body as having a 'flow' of grotesque, foul-smelling, dark 'stuff' leaving it and falling down to the floor because it is heavy. All the senses are involved in the method and you must not only smell, feel and see but also hear the vile stuff leaving the body, using all your imagination and ingenuity to make the energy-stuff 'real'. This visualisation is practised for about five minutes a day. About a week or so after I began the experiment, my wart showed no sign of change so I stopped. A few days later it seemed that the wart was a little smaller but I took no notice, thinking it was my imagination. But within a week the wart had completely gone. Though I cannot say that 'healing energy' was responsible, I am in no doubt that the visualisation and focus for five minutes a day was the 'active agent' in eliminating the wart. Qi may work in a similar way but in reverse, as a *positive* energy flow guided by intent. If we use our intent to focus on particular parts of the body, blood will flow there and we can say that Qi follows in much the same way as the 'dirty energy' flowed out of my wart. When we perform Jiangan we can be aware of the positive Qi energy entering our bodies and giving us vibrant health and well-being as it flows through us. We can focus on a particular part of the body as we exercise and the blood will follow the intent and flow there. Is this Qi? Whether Qi is responsible for the well-being and health we may attain from practice of Chinese internal arts and traditional Chinese medicine is a profound question which we cannot answer as yet.

FOLLOWING IN THE SUCCESS OF TAIJI

Taiji has been subjected to a great deal of research since the 1970s and has been shown to be beneficial for many health problems. I believe that Jiangan could also be successful in similar areas as it has greater health promotion potential. One of the high-profile medical conditions where Taiji has made a difference is combating falls in elderly people. Jiangan can make a contribution in this respect by improving the strength and muscle tone of legs through its safe squats and lunges with the weight distributed on both legs equally. This is especially important for elderly people, who may have weak knees. Taiji also teaches good body alignment and mental focus. Jiangan, being simpler to learn and practise, would offer many patients an alternative and safe route to developing these qualities.

FOLLOWING IN THE SUCCESS OF QIGONG

Qigong (sometimes written as Chi Kung), meaning breath or energy work, is probably the closest 'relative' to Jiangan. In recent years it has become increasingly popular in the West and throughout the world. Although as an art it is difficult to define, essentially Qigong is a term used to describe various methods of health training developed in China, predominantly utilising breathing techniques. Although Qi can relate to 'energy', it is more ambiguous and wide-ranging. It shows the relationship between matter, energy and spirit, but in the context of breathing exercises Qigong tends to mean cultivating the body's energy. Breathing is always involved so Qi is strongly linked with breath and life force. The earliest Qigong was influenced by Daoist philosophy but branched out to various schools including medical, Confucionist, Buddhist and martial arts. It can be further split into different methods such as static (sitting or standing in one posture) and dynamic (slow moving forms much like Taiji, which are the most popular routines practised today). Qigong has a rich history stretching back thousands of years and contains much of the wisdom of traditional Chinese medicine. Many of these ancient routines are still taught today, including 'Muscle and Tendon Strengthening' exercise, 'Five Animals Frolics' and 'Eight Treasures', though they have frequently been adapted in the twentieth century. There are new Qigong routines being devised and 'resurrected' from the past by committees of Qigong specialists in China. Jiangan can certainly be regarded as Qigong in the broadest sense, but its methodology is quite different from the mainstream and popularly practised Qigong routines, which indicates a separate development. But all the wonderful health benefits that have been observed from the practice of the popular Qigong routines can certainly be obtained from Jiangan, even if Jiangan works the body in a more general way and does not target specific meridians like Qigong. The medical literature on positive effects of Qigong is growing, and there is no doubt that Jiangan can also make a contribution in this area. The fact that Jiangan's methodology is significantly different from modern Qigong with its aesthetic flowing circular movements may concern some 'purists' who have studied only popular Qigong. But medical trials have shown that a wide variety of breathing exercises can be effective. In Russia, conditions such as pulmonary tuberculosis and asthma were successfully treated with the 'Buteyko' breathing method, which also brought marked improvement of symptoms in patients suffering from more serious conditions such as radiation sickness and HIV. In India, Yoga-type breathing has also proven effective in a wide range of conditions. Within Qigong itself there are hundreds of widely differing styles, including ancient methods rather like Yoga that have been shown to produce beneficial effects. This shows that the 'active ingredient' of breathing exercises is the breathing itself rather than a style of movement. The significant advantage of Jiangan over popular Qigong is that an entire routine produces over 100 beneficial (deep diaphragmatic) breathing cycles because of the graduated stages. But with repetitions this figure can rise to over 300. As most of these breathing cycles occur during the graduated stages leading up to the final Yang posture, there is less strain on the body than having one breathing cycle for the entire posture and repeating that posture several times.

10

Guide to Practice

INTEGRATION WITH EASTERN ARTS CLASSES

Although Jiangan is effective on many levels and it is perfectly possible to practise it as a mind-body system in its own right, those studying Chinese martial arts will receive particular benefit and find that it is a structured, time-honoured, safe, comprehensive basis for stretching and strengthening, as well as offering historical and philosophical consistency – in short, a perfect companion to the Chinese internal arts. Taiji and Qigong classes usually begin with a set of warm-ups consisting of 'loosening' circling movements. One of the beneficial aspects of Taiji is the way it employs circular movements in its forms, but using circular movements to loosen joints frequently causes practitioners to use momentum which can cause strains. Circular movements in warm-ups are also rather repetitive and psychologically limiting because they are frequently carried out in an automatic fashion. They are regarded as separate to the main exercises of the class – a means to an end before the 'real' mind-body work begins.

With Jiangan for warm-ups we move only one part of the body or muscle group in one direction at a time. This gives more control and reduces the chance of strains from multidirectional forces. The Gan ensures slowness, consistency and stability, gives Qi energy awareness, requires hand-tasking and employs mindfulness. This integrated approach provides intent and focus that is a strong link between warm-ups and the main exercises of the class.

Of particular interest for the Taiji practitioner is the fact that Jiangan offers significant exercises for the arms and the upper body. This makes it an ideal companion to Taiji, which works the legs extremely well but lacks arm-strengthening exercises. I always begin my Taiji classes with the standing exercises as these are adequate to gently limber up the body for Taiji. But anyone running a martial art class of any tradition – in fact anyone running classes of any physical discipline – can benefit from the stretching, strengthening and gentle opening up Jiangan provides.

INTERNAL AND GENTLE

Because the Gan is made from a hard substance, many people are intimidated by it and assume that the exercises are physical or superficial. This is understandable because most exercises that use implements are very physical in nature. But Jiangan develops the body from within to achieve a truly healthy and balanced body. To produce external results it must first be approached as an internal exercise with the correct attitude. There should be no tension, either physical or mental. Most people are aware of physical tension especially in muscles but mental tension is often overlooked. It is frequently caused by approaching something with a little too much solemnity or enthusiasm for getting details just right. Internal health systems demand not only 'control' and 'focus' but also 'letting go', and achieving a balance between these two states is the secret of mastery. Too much focus creates a heavy mindset which actually defeats an important part of the internal arts – to relax body and mind. Jiangan movements are subtle and originate from stillness and are led by breathing. Your movements should be both relaxed and precise (letting go and control simultaneously). And just like in Taiji, 'relaxed' does not mean 'floppy' or slouching. We stand erect with no tension because it is not a 'physical' exercise. There are some important pointers on maintaining this internal spirit. When the Gan is in contact with the back of your shoulders, for example, it must always sit lightly. Never 'rest' your hands heavily on the Gan so that it digs down against your shoulders. If you feel that the Gan has become heavy, rest and return to the exercise later. *Gentle persistence brings reward.* When your arms and upper body are sufficiently strengthened, you will be able to hold the Gan in the correct position for longer while supporting it with your arms. Using a Gan that is too thick or heavy will hamper your progress and block your quest for the internal spirit of the art.

PERSONAL EMPOWERMENT FOR HEALTH

The refreshing difference between Jiangan and other internal exercise systems is that lessons are not really needed and teachers are unnecessary as long as you can follow the authentic instructions. That does not mean that you would not benefit from personal face-to-face instruction, but many people, including myself, have learnt Jiangan from a book. Anyone with a reasonable degree of insight and intelligence can learn from written instructions. The hypothesis that a potent and safe ancient health system can be practised by anyone without recourse to lessons or a teacher is empowering.

RAPID BENEFITS

Because Jiangan targets, stretches and strengthens essential muscles effectively, you will notice the effects after about a week of daily practice. After several weeks your legs will feel stronger, your hip joints looser and your back muscles noticeably toned. And if you have extra pounds, you will certainly experience a reduction and shaping of muscles in that area.

MEDITATION

Jiangan is a form of moving meditation. The focus is on intentional movement and deep breathing, feeling your body being gently exercised. This means that Jiangan is not a chore to get through like conventional exercises. Like Taiji, the physical movements are 'dead' until we bring them alive with our mind. The body is like a train set. Our will (conscious intent) is the electricity and when the current is switched off the train must stop. So we must become *attentive to every movement and every breath*. If the mind wanders we must stop moving because the intent is lost. You should practise the 17 Exercises Routine gracefully, slowly, with focus and dignity. Then you will discover that Jiangan is anything but boring. Interest is maintained by tangible goals as the Gan works its way to set positions and we can focus on maintaining correct posture, breathing, awareness of pyramid energy circulation, Qi energy flow and healing using visualisation if necessary. You do not have to be aware of any of these things or all of them at the same time, but certainly the Gan can become a focus for our energy and intent in a way that could take some people to metaphysical heights (so 'Wand' in the magical sense is an apt English translation for the Gan).

The graduated stages methodology is the key to maintaining interest; there is a target, a definite aim and intent to reach your own Yang position and eventually improve it. This provides a sense of progress and purpose in your exercises, which is psychologically invaluable.

Getting the Focus Right

'Attention', 'focus', 'concentration', 'letting go', 'emptying the mind': many concepts have been used to describe the mental state during meditation. So what should we think about during Jiangan practice? First, we must not concentrate. Concentration is focused attention. This can be useful for performing some detailed tasks but it has one big drawback; it drains our other senses and prevents our minds from processing a wide range of input. For example, someone deeply absorbed in an interesting book or fascinating magazine article may have to be called several times before he or she 'hears' the caller. Pickpockets distract their victims by intensifying their focus on another part of their body or on an incident, thereby overshadowing the victims' sense of touch so that they do not feel their watch being taken from their wrist. Therefore focused attention – concentration – takes away our sensitivity to the world around us. This is not the type of mental state conducive to the practice of moving meditation. We need constant input from the senses and our surroundings. Beginners will often concentrate when learning movements and so block out these essential signals.

The opposite of concentration is non-focus or 'emptying the mind'. This is the state often wrongly attributed to meditation. In fact it is difficult, if not impossible, to empty the mind because it can never really be 'empty'; we always have to be aware of 'something' during waking consciousness. Still, it is possible not be attentive to anything in particular and let the mind drift. The common misconception is that meditation involves this type of 'empty' mental state but the opposite is true. Meditation is being aware of *something*.

The prime danger of trying to empty the mind is that the mind and body separate and fragmentation occurs. Paying attention to what we are doing is an essential part of Chinese internal arts, whether Taiji, Qigong or Jiangan, and once we lose that awareness then our movements become meaningless and we go into 'automatic pilot' mode just like changing gears while driving a car. This leads to bad habits.

So how can this be prevented? It is obvious that a middle ground is desirable; neither concentration nor empty-mindedness is conducive to moving meditation. In the face of practising moments we know by heart, we need to maintain a light 'grip' on our awareness of our body and surroundings. This state is rather like the analogy of the infant's grasp that is neither too tight nor weak – the way we grasp the Gan. Environmental factors influence mental states, especially with beginners. Practising alone it is easy to relax one's focus and let the mind drift, whereas practising with a group or in public we are sometimes so focused that we become unaware of external stimuli. The first time I took part in a group Taiji display in front of a crowd of people, my teacher later told me that I was drifting all over the place. This was something I never did in class but my focus during the display veered towards concentration and I was simply unaware of my distancing. To help avoid both these extremes, if practising in public imagine you are practising alone, and when practising alone imagine a group of people watching you. You will eventually achieve the 'middle ground' so that wherever and however you practise, your focus will be balanced.

The Liberating Prison

Moving meditation often expands the consciousness, while many sitting meditating nirvana-seekers are left disappointed. The secret is that in giving attention to simple movements the conscious mind is doing what it does best – working within limitation. One's unconscious is freed and works in parallel to bring up occasional insights of great profundity and feelings of peace and wholeness where everything fits in place. So without striving for enlightenment we expand our consciousness within the limitations of a moving form. The set movements of a form may be a 'prison' but it is a prison that ultimately liberates the spirit. Those sitting in meditation are confronted with a wide plane of emptiness because they have little to focus on so there is a danger of wandering thoughts and emotions. This is why practitioners of sitting meditation are taught to focus on their breathing or a specific thought or point; it creates a 'form' that the conscious mind can understand.

There is a wonderful poem in Lao Zi's *Dao de Jing* for the concept of becoming free within limitation:

> *Without going out of the door we can know the World,*
> *without looking out of the window we can know the way of heaven.*

The Three Treasures 三 寶

Although Daoist meditation techniques are beyond the scope of this book, the simplest way to describe the process is through 'The Three Treasures'. These are concepts of traditional Chinese medicine and internal arts which originate from Daoist thought. The name 'Three Treasures' (sanbao 三寶) reflects their importance within Daoist arts, although concepts and practices associated with the terms are complex and vary in meaning according to the context.

- Jing (body) 精
- Qi (energy) 氣
- Shen (spirit) 神

Jing corresponds to the body, Qi to energy and Shen to spirit or the soul. Applying these terms to moving meditation simply means that when the movements become natural to you, you become aware of your body and how it is moving (Jing stage). Many people will not want to go beyond this stage but others will eventually shift awareness during their practice to how the movements are affecting energies within their body (Qi stage). Those who want to go further can become aware of more subtle and refined energy not only within them but also surrounding them, which encompasses 'essence', 'aura' or 'spirit' (Shen stage). After practising for some time, you may feel a process of transformation taking place on all three levels. This is a type of *inner alchemy* and can be attested to by people who practise Chinese internal arts such as Taiji and Qigong as well as many forms of meditation and Yoga.

They transform into more positive, happier and contented people. Achieving Shen or spirit is the goal of balanced meditation.

Meditation on Qi

You can envisage Qi entering the hands through the Gan when you inhale and feel it go along the length of the Gan and up the arms into the body, down to the Dan Tian and then down to the Huiyin point under the base of the spine. While exhaling you can envisage Qi raising from the Huiyin point to the Baihui point at the crown of the head. Qi is always circulated around the body and some goes down the arms to the Gan to be recirculated and some of it travels to whichever part of the body is focused upon.

Visualisation

Meditation can help encourage the body to heal itself and even improve physical strength and stamina. The mind leads and the body follows. Stories of elderly women lifting vehicles that have trapped their sons have become the stuff of urban legend but in moments of crisis our bodies really are capable of amazing feats of strength and endurance. Visualisation can change the way the body reacts to external surroundings and stress. One day when I was about 12 years old, I was running home across the school playing fields when I noticed that the exit seemed a very long way away. I got out of breath and my legs felt very heavy and tiredness swept over me. I slowed down – but suddenly I had the vision of a football on the ground a few feet in front of me. My instinct was to kick it 'mentally' but the ball was just a little too far away so I tried to catch it. My legs suddenly felt light and I was no longer breathless. I made the ball disappear and immediately I felt tired and my legs were as heavy as lead once again. So I deliberately brought the ball back and began chasing it and felt light and energised. Again I made the imaginary ball disappear and saw only an expanse of field in front of me; almost immediately my lungs were heavy and my legs could no longer keep up at the pace I was running, and I had to slow down immediately. I repeated this exercise several times and each time I chased the ball, I became energised and each time it disappeared I was out of breath and my legs were heavy. Without knowing it I had discovered the power of visualisation.

A similar thing happened to me some years later when I was working as a hospital porter and had to carry heavy rubbish bags down from the top floor of an old four-storey house with no lift. If I tried to take the bag down the narrow flights of stairs in one go, I would have to put it down to rest once or twice on a landing. On one occasion, approaching a landing, I thought of putting the bag down to rest and immediately the bag felt lighter and I could move much more easily. Intrigued, I did not put the bag down but continued descending and passed by the landing; the bag instantly felt heavier. Then, approaching the next landing I convinced myself that I was going to put the bag down again; as soon as that idea came to me the bag again seemed less heavy. I got to the ground floor without putting the bag down once to rest. What was happening? Without a target or aim, the mind collapses into a sort of hopelessness and the body 'gives up'. Positive visualisation on a tangible target is essential not only for psychological well-being but also for self healing. So practising visualisation while performing Jiangan can increase its beneficial effects.

RELAXATION

Relaxation is essential during Jiangan. Many people want to relax but do not know how. Relaxation is important yet it can be elusive. If we 'try' to relax, we are reacting only to an intangible word that means nothing if you are tense. The mind needs practical help on how to relax and Jiangan provides this with form, precise method and focus. As you perform the exercises correctly and become aware of the important points, relaxation will follow eventually – especially if you pay attention to your breathing.

LISTENING TO YOUR BODY

It is common, after a round of Taiji, Yoga or Qigong, for the long-term practitioner to experience a warm glow in his or her muscles, especially in the back region, as if it is tingling with energy. This pleasant 'afterglow' is a factor of all internal exercises because they work the body gently; there is no exhaustion, tiredness or traumatised body parts. After Jiangan's 17 Exercises Routine this pleasing feeling can be felt to a heightened degree because the body has been worked in a more targeted, scientific yet still gentle way. The most pleasing phenomenon is felt beginning a particular exercise after the preceding one has worked muscles in a particular way, as if the new direction of movement is complementing the previous exercise and the muscles are warmly 'welcoming' the change of direction. This is felt particularly strongly between adjacent exercises such as:

- 'Peeling the Octopus' and 'Twisting the Snake'

- 'Twisting the Snake' and 'Twitching the Dragon's Tail'

- 'Tailor's Walk' and 'Rolling the Panda'.

The comfortable feeling in the muscles during these 'pairings' (as if a particular problem is being solved) provides the body with a sense of completion and is evidence of the system's scientific and logical sequence.

Not all parts of the body respond in the same way to the exercises. The human body is not perfectly proportioned and symmetrical and some people will have a weakness in the right or left side. This can be felt when performing exercises such as 'Twitching the Dragon's Tail'. In the 'twist' you may find it easier to reach the ideal Yang position on either the right or the left side. Accept this and do not try to force one side of the body to 'compete' with the other, but simply go as far as is comfortable on each side. I find it easier to reach the Yang stage on the left side than the right in that particular exercise. The same applies to exercises that require you to work one leg then the other, such as the penultimate exercise, 'Dragon Kicks'. Here I cannot lift my left leg as high as my right but this is the natural state of my body and so I raise it only as far as is comfortable. The same applies to any exercise in the routine, either standing or floor exercises.

MUSIC

It is especially pleasing for our mood to exercise to music or atmospheric sounds. But we should choose the right kind of music to match our style of exercise. Studies have shown that the faster the tempo of music played during exercise, the more physically robust we tend to become and the faster our heart works. The beats per minute (bpm) of rock, pop and dance music are suited to more energetic exercise and so 'high energy fitness music', 'aerobic music' and 'workout music' has evolved, which makes energetic exercise more efficient. But music for internal health exercises such as Taiji, Qigong, Yoga and Jiangan needs to be in tune with the calm movements, deep breathing and slower heart rate. I personally have found that listening to uplifting classical pieces such as the 'The Lark Ascending' by Ralph Vaughan Williams is very conducive to meditation exercise. The profound and uplifting nature of such music provides emotional and psychological support in tune with the meditative aims of the exercises. The music genres labelled 'new age', 'ambient' or 'space music', typified by groups like Tangerine Dream, also encourage a meditative frame of mind and help us to get into the mood of internal exercises. Traditional Chinese music – particularly solo bamboo flute pieces – provides an especially good environment for Jiangan and is also an excellent choice for accompanying moving meditation.

Music has profound effects on the human psyche that go beyond providing a 'mood' for exercise class. It can also add a genuinely healing element to internal exercises. As discussed in Chapter 4, maintaining balance between 'Yin Qi' and 'Yang Qi' is an important concept in traditional Chinese medicine. If we regard the vibration of music as a manifestation of Qi this will have ramifications on how our choice of music affects our body, especially during exercises. If we follow this principle then just as Yang Qi stimulates the body, Yang music stimulates the mind and spirit, which in turn energises the body. Yang is heaven and movement so it is important to have rhythm, syncopation and foot-tapping elements with drums and beats. Throughout history this type of music was used to rouse warriors for fighting and to accompany dancing. Although such music is thought 'primitive' and 'primal', if we follow Chinese philosophy it is Yin music which came first. Yin is earth and stillness, and just as Yin Qi cools down the body, Yin music helps us to unwind and relax. An example of Yin music is a piece that offers uplifting, static or slow-moving agreeable harmonies and which contains a sense of uplifting 'otherworldliness'; Yin music is frequently used for meditation and contemplation.

Looked at in this way, it is important that humans receive a healthy daily 'diet' of both Yin and Yang music to remain physiologically balanced because both fundamental sources of musical vibration are present in the human psyche. When practising Jiangan, Yin music helps relax us, calms the mind and puts us in the mood to pay attention to the movements. The 'genre' of music we use is not important as long as the Yin element is represented to a significant degree. Unfortunately, a huge amount of commercial 'popular' music seems to have detached itself from both Yin and Yang sources and neither uplifts nor stimulates. Bland music of this type corresponds to highly processed food and so consequently most people are in a state of 'musical-emotional scurvy', starved of psychological benefit offered by the two ancient sources of music vibration. My own daily musical diet consists of relaxing Yin music (such as Gregorian chant or traditional Japanese Shakuhachi flute music) to meditate and practise Jiangan, and energising Yang music (dance music such as Trance or Techno) when I feel in need of a 'lift'. The importance of music in psychological health cannot be underestimated. Tones with certain regular intervals are very harmonious to humans whereas 'noise' – that is, random or irregular patterns – annoys, upsets and disturbs us. Animals, plants and even bacteria are affected by music vibrations (bacteria multiply voraciously under the influence of certain frequencies and are killed when subjected to others). So it is a little easier to understand how with certain chants and 'healing tones', the ancients could treat illnesses within the body.

THE MOZART OF EXERCISE

Simplicity is the key to mastering Jiangan.

The piano music of Franz List is brilliant, technically difficult and contains an overwhelming variety of content. But only virtuoso pianists can really play these pieces. The piano music of Mozart is comparatively simple, yet this simplicity ensures that the average pianist has a chance to play it. Limitation of technique is often deceptive and hides a profundity of comprehensive content while being more accessible. Jiangan's simple methodology is a little like this. A complex exercise can be a drawback for the average person who simply wants to keep fit or maintain health with a simple daily regime. For the average person to be confronted by a myriad of specialist exercises is essentially 'overkill'.

People may go to the gym to lose weight, attend aerobics classes to trim their abdominals and stomachs and attend Taiji, Qigong and Yoga classes to calm their mind from the tension of hectic modern life and to become more supple. This fragmented approach can be both expensive and time-consuming for those looking for a simple and effective daily exercise. If the average person wants the benefits of internal and external exercise in one simple comprehensive routine, Jiangan is the perfect exercise. Another significant comparison with Mozart piano music is that it is easy for people of different levels to get what they seek. In the same way that a concert pianist and an amateur will both be able to play the music and will get something different out of it, with Jiangan a very fit athlete can practise Jiangan aiming for the ideal postures and doing many repetitions while an unfit elderly person can practise it much more cautiously and gently alongside the athlete.

THE SECULAR GAN

After exploring the philosophical background of Jiangan, it may seem contradictory to state that the art is essentially secular and practical, not esoteric and spiritual. But the art was not meant for people who wanted to explore esoteric concepts, perform specialist healing or gain spiritual insights. It is aimed at simply promoting good general health for the average person. The philosophical background to the art is not essential for progress and you can certainly practise Jiangan without knowledge of it. So those who have an aversion to the philosophical and esoteric ideas of ancient China for whatever reason can practise Jiangan on a purely practical and physical basis and obtain equally successful results.

RESPECT

The master–apprentice (or teacher–student) relationship goes deep into the human psyche and has stood the test of time. That the student should accept what the teacher prescribes sounds obvious but many students in the West have a strong 'client' mentality that undermines the teaching process. Clients not only know exactly what they want to learn but also want to dictate the methods by which they learn it. This results in a pick-and-mix mentality and a lack of respect not only for the teacher but also for the art and all those who have gone before. In Jiangan when students encounter a difficult section, some may want to perform it in their own way or even miss the section out altogether. This is a lack of respect for not only the instructor but also the art and all the previous generations who accumulated knowledge only to have it discarded at a whim. I mention this in case any reader is tempted to make significant changes to the exercises or the whole routine.

Following 隨

I believe that it is highly significant that 17 exercises were chosen for the daily routine and that this number may be linked to the *Yi Jing* (known in the West as *I Ching, The Book of Changes*), one of the oldest Chinese classic texts. This book contains a divination system but many scholars agree that it has far-reaching psychological and metaphysical implications. It is primarily a book advising humans on the correct behaviour to adopt under various conditions. There are 64 'Hexagrams', which are complex arrangements of 'Yin' and 'Yang' lines. Hexagram number 17 is 'Sui' 隨, which means 'following'. The pronouncement accompanying this particular hexagram is 'The path of following correctly leads to development and great success'

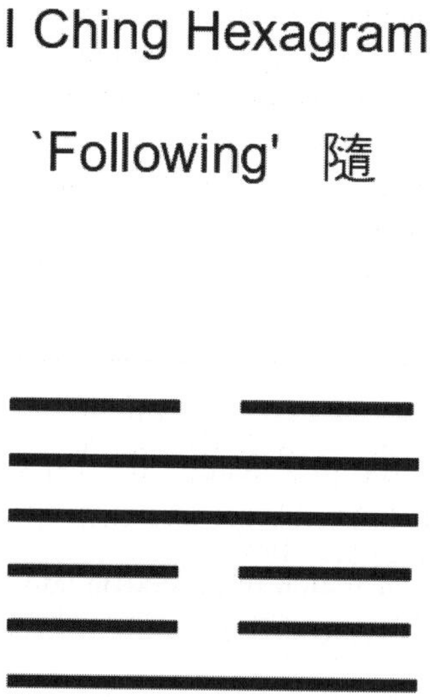

I Ching Hexagram 17

`Following' 隨

Figure XVI

which indicates that students will meet great success but only if they follow instructions correctly. Figure XVI shows the hexagram.

Protecting the Legacy

Eastern arts such as Yoga, Taiji and Qigong have many styles and schools and many different variations of postures and routines. Two practitioners of different styles will often say something like, 'We practise this posture quite differently to you.' Jiangan does not follow this model and should never do so because it has evolved not through branching out into many different styles but by being focused into the most efficient methodology. The challenge in this age of instant communication is ensuring that 'One Hundred Schools' do *not* bloom in Jiangan. The specific methodologies were devised because all other methodologies *did not work or were not safe*. This point cannot be stressed too strongly. Jiangan did not develop different 'styles' like other internal arts simply because of this simple physiological reality. The danger is that as a result of increased popularity, there may be different forms springing up that do not follow the methodology handed down to us that is proven safe and effective. This is not a matter of being dictatorial or intolerant of different 'styles', but simply protecting methodology that works and is known to be safe. Taking an analogy from mathematics, if a particular problem was solved by a fifteenth-century mathematician, it is solved. Period. Because the line of continuous evolution in Jiangan has been lost, the only way to ensure safe and effective methodology is to follow the instructions from previous generations. This means that every practitioner must have free and open access to the source text. If we rely only upon attending classes and following teachers, there is a risk that we fall victim to the 'Chinese whispers syndrome'. There will be Jiangan teachers who employ methodology that Johnson expressly warned against, because nobody is perfect and we can all go astray and forget certain points. This is precisely why every student needs open access to the source text so that they can diligently study it. This will prevent the gradual sloppy deterioration of the exercises.

Any changes made to the exercises either by an individual or group at this time will lead to the detriment of the art. We may have to wait for many centuries before further changes are made. There is every reason to be patient.